Thinking about losing weight

How I lost 40 pounds in 40 days
and you can too
Help, Hints & Hacks
for weight loss
40 pounds = 18 kilograms

**Author James A. Love
(A.K.A 'The Irish Guru')**

Thinking About Losing Weight

****

Copyright © 2018 James A Love

All rights reserved. No part of this book may be reproduced in any form or by any electronic or mechanical means, including information storage and retrieval systems, without permission in writing from the publisher, except by reviewers, who may quote brief passages in a review.

ISBN-13: 9781717855954

Published by Saints & Scholars Publishing

Contact - help@irishguru.com   Visit www.irishguru.com

The information contained in this book is intended to be educational and not for diagnosis, prescription, or treatment of any health disorder whatsoever. This book is written with the understanding that neither the author nor publisher is engaged in rendering any medical or psychological advice. Readers should consult their physician prior to beginning a new exercise program, changing their diet, quitting smoking, or making other lifestyle changes. The publisher and author disclaim personal liability, directly or indirectly, for the information presented within.

****

DEDICATION

I owe this book to my family who I love with all my heart.
Thank you for all your help and support on my weight loss
journey particularly to my daughter Abigail who never
doubted my ability. Also to my faithful dog Delilah who
enjoyed and sometimes endured the many long walks.

CONTENTS

Introduction 7

Day 1 – The Big Why? 9

Day 2 - Seeing the thin you 14

Day 3 - The Yo-Yo Craze 18

Day 4 - Uisce beatha – The water of Life 21

Day 5 - Good Night 25

Day 6 - The times they are a-changing 28

Day 7 - Get moving 32

Day 8 – Back to nature 36

Day 9 - Do you have an ADDICTION? 40

Day 10 - Pass the sugar, please 44

Day 11 - Which diet is the best? 48

Day 12 – Eat yourself thin 52

Day 13 – Go with your gut 56

Day 14 – Take time to Chew 60

Day 15 – The long night 64

Day 16 – Skip a day 68

Day 17 - Stressed out 72

Thinking About Losing Weight

Day 18 - Tricks of the Mind   76

Day 19 – Technology and weight loss   79

Day 20 – 4 steps to confidence   82

Day 21 – Halfway Mark   86

Day 22 – Breathe   88

Day 23 – Greek Yogurt   90

Day 24 – An apple a Day   92

Day 25 – Weigh yourself   94

Day 26 – Rise and Shine   96

Day 27 – Lift something heavy   98

Day 28 – What colour is your tea?   100

Day 29 – The hunger game   102

Day 30 – Go Nuts   104

Day 31 - Motivate yourself   106

Day 32 – Diet Drinks   108

Day 33 – Sprint   110

Day 34 – Prepare your own food   112

Day 35 – Eat fat to lose fat   114

Day 36 – Focus on being healthy rather than thin 116

Day 37 – You can do it! Learned helplessness   118

Day 38 – You can do it! Self-efficacy   120

Day 39 – You are amazing   122

Day 40 – The last laugh   124

INTRODUCTION

You can lose 40 pounds in 40 days. I know because I did it. 47 years of age and fat. After 17 years of slowly piling on a pound here and a pound there, going up a waist size this year and another a few years later, I found myself classified as obese. It was time for decisive action.

I had the knowledge, the books on the shelf from the '4 Hour Body' (Tim Ferris) to 'You are what you eat' (Gillian McKeith) and every variation in-between. Amazingly having these books and even reading these books had no effect on my waistline. I had to move from knowledge to action and that is what this book is all about. The motivation to just do it. Helping you move from aspirations to actually accomplishing your goals.

It is your time to start the journey from thinking "I need to lose some weight," to actually doing something about it. Leave behind the worn out mantra, "I will begin my diet tomorrow" for we all know that tomorrow never comes. Change it to "In 40 days or 4 months I will weigh xxx lbs" and then go for it. Set your goal, draw up your plan and begin to lose those pounds.

I wish I could be with you as your personal coach, cheering you along the way, but through these pages, I will walk beside you in your journey giving you the daily motivation that you need to become the weight that you desire to be. This book is not a how-to method or a step to step guide; it is more the voice of a friend encouraging you to do the best that you can. I want you to see those visible changes in your body, feel your health level rise and for you to be the best version of you that you can be.

"Your body is the baggage you must carry through life. The more excess the baggage, the shorter the trip."
Arnold H. Glasgow

Footnotes:
This is not a diet book or diet plan there are plenty of those out there. Your shelves are probably already full of them.

This is not a scientific study and you should talk to your doctor or dietitian to help you determine your specific calorie needs for weight loss. Most overweight men and women may be able to safely lose 40 pounds limiting intake to 1,200 to 1,600 calories a day, according to the National Heart, Lung and Blood Institute.

Disclaimer - None of the advice contained in this book is to be considered as medical advice. Please do not make any changes to your lifestyle without discussing it with your doctor. The intent of the author is to convey personal experience in the hope that it may be of help in others' personal quests for permanent weight loss and the eradication of overeating. The author shall in no event be held liable to any party for any direct, indirect, punitive, special, incidental or other consequential damages arising directly or indirectly from any use of this material, which is provided "as is" and without warranties. This book is not intended to treat, cure, or prevent any disease or illness. This information is intended for educational purposes only, not as medical advice. Always check with your doctor before changing your diet, eating, or health program.

Day 1 – The Big Why?

Weight loss is not a physical challenge. It's a mental one.

Find your why? Losing weight is about so much more than diets and workouts. We need to discover our deep motivation to get and stay thin.

This is true: when you have determined in your mind your deep motivation for getting and staying thin, sticking to a diet or workout plan stops feeling like a daily battle. Weight loss becomes easier and being thin becomes part of your core identity.

I need to ask you right at the start of this journey that we are walking together: What is your reason for losing weight? Isn't that obvious you think, I want to be thin. But I need to probe your thinking a little bit more. Why my friend, why do you want to be thin? After all, you have perhaps wanted to be thin for many years and nothing about your lifestyle, diet or body shape has changed. In order for you to achieve your goal, it's important to dig a little deeper and find your true motivation.

Is it your family? You used to be able to keep up easily with the children now they can outrun you. You don't want your teenage son or daughter to be embarrassed to be seen with you. Maybe it's your own health. You're getting sick and tired of being sick and tired. Granddad or dad died of heart disease, cancer or some other weight related illness and now you are at the stage of life that you are no longer feeling invincible and have decided to do something about it. You want to not just be alive, but looking fabulous at your children's wedding. You have to provide for your family or achieve your great aims in life. You want to be able to play football with the grandchildren... and so we could go on. You need a WHY that is deep and strong to give you the motivation to keep going when it seems that everything is screaming at you, GIVE UP, PIG OUT, FEED YOUR FACE. You need a motivation that will keep you on track when the pressure from within and without is to quit.

This chapter is where we do the hard work. Pen, paper and honesty are needed as we work through it together. Studies have shown that when you put pen to paper, you make your brain say, "Hey, something important is happening. I better pay attention!"

So take your paper and pen and do this exercise. This is so important that you don't skip over this. This exercise, called Seven Levels Deep, is used by American consultant Joe Stump with his high-level clients. Many of us have a why that originated in our heads, not our hearts. Quite often we have whys we adopted from other people because they sounded good to us. The idea of Seven Levels Deep is to ask seven consecutive questions. Each question naturally leads to the next question, but you have to do it seven times. Not three. Not five. Not nine. Seven. The purpose is to cut through the layers of whys we form in our head, and get deep to the core of our being for what truly motivates us. It gets to the heart of our why. This paper exercise is foundational for all that is to come. Write down this question then answer it. What is your reason for losing weight? Now we need to take it a little further and deeper. Write this next question and answer it also. Why is this important to you? Keep asking this question "Why is this important to you?" until you reach your seventh answer. Give it a go and see how far, how deep you can go.

This is the real WHY behind your reason for wanting to lose weight and it is different for everyone but you must find it to give you the motivation to keep going and achieve your weight loss goal. The deeper your WHY, the more motivated you will be and the more likely you are to succeed.

Set your goal! Once you have found your motivation, you need to set achievable realistic goals. I am suggesting that you follow the guidelines of SMART goals. This will lead to a goal that is specific, measurable, achievable, relevant and time-bound. It's a great way to set goals that have meaning and purpose. Dare I say it's even a "smart" way to set a goal? If you take just ten minutes to walk through this process you'll start losing weight with more confidence and direction. So get your paper and pen and let's get writing.

Specific - Avoid setting goals that are too broad. A broad goal goes something like – "I want to lose weight for the summer holidays." You need to refine your goal into a specific milestone that you'd like to reach. One way to help refine your goal is to speak to your doctor. If you are considering weight loss, your doctor may be able to tell you how losing a certain amount of weight will improve your health. Or consult a weight loss chart, work out what your ideal weight should be and see how much you need to lose in order to reach that target. Then your specific goal becomes – "I want to lose 30 pounds before I go on my summer holidays."

Measurable - In order to track your progress during the weight loss journey, the goal you set needs to be measurable. In our weight loss journey, the scales will measure our progress. Our adjusted goal becomes – "I want to lose 30 pounds before I go on my summer holidays. I will measure my weight on the scale to track my progress."

Attainable - To make your weight loss goal attainable, you should evaluate your past history losing weight. If you've never been able to lose more than ten pounds, then a weight loss goal of 30 pounds might not be reasonable. Remember that once you reach a goal, you can always set a new one. All goals should be challenging but they shouldn't be so difficult that they are overwhelming. Adjust your goal so that it is reasonable. "I want to lose 20 pounds before I go on my summer holidays. I will measure my weight on the scale to track my progress. When I reach 20 pounds, I will re-evaluate and consider setting a new goal for continued weight loss."

Relevant - Your goal needs to matter in your life. Defining why the goal matters may help you stay motivated when complacency sets in. This is where you add in your WHY. Define how weight loss is relevant in your life and remind yourself of these reasons when you are tempted to give up. Your adjusted resolution becomes - "I want to lose 20 pounds before I go on my summer holidays. I will measure my weight on the scale to track my progress. When I reach 20 pounds, I will re-evaluate and consider setting a new goal for continued weight loss. Losing this weight will mean _ _ _ _ _ _ (Here you add your WHY)"

Time-Bound - Each resolution should have a time limit. That is, you should decide on a reasonable amount of time that you'll take to reach your goal. For weight loss, keep in mind that a 1-2 pound loss a week is generally considered reasonable, although short periods of quick weight loss can be used by dieters as well. For our purpose, we are setting ourselves a time limit of 40 days. So work out when you are going to start, get the date of 40 days ahead and set that as your time.

Go for it - Now that you have your goal.
Super **SMART** goal – "I want to lose 20 pounds by (date 40 days from now). I will measure my weight on the scale to track my progress. I will weigh (enter your target weight) When I reach 20 pounds, I will re-evaluate and consider setting a new goal for continued weight loss. Losing this weight will mean _ _ _ _ _ _ (Here you add your **WHY**)"

   I want you to write it down on an index card. Carry that index card around with you and read it whenever you need motivation. You don't feel like exercising? Read that index card. The office vending machine is tempting you? Read that index card. Read it first thing in the morning. Read it before you go to bed. Make copies and put it up wherever it makes sense: on the fridge, the bathroom mirror, at the office. Wherever you can.

"Only I can change my life. No one can do it for me."
                        Carol Burnett

DAY 2 - SEEING THE THIN YOU

"Doubt Kills More Dreams Than Failure Ever Will"
Suzy Kassem

My friend was struggling with a weight problem continually trying so hard to diet. One night she was visiting friends who had kindly made a big supper. (In Ireland supper is food eaten late in the evening that we have no need to eat but is often part of a social occasion.) She politely tried to decline but the host replied, "I know a big girl like you can eat plenty, eat up." And so she did as she was told and ate up. Do you have an inner voice that is telling you to eat up? It is not in the scope of this book to discern where that voice might be coming from but instead to replace it with a new voice.

It is a known fact that thoughts and emotions affect the body for better or worse, depending on your predominant thoughts and emotions. Negative thinking, stress, fear, excitement, worry and anger hurt the body. Under these conditions, the body releases toxins into the blood, which affect it adversely. Positive thinking, happiness, love and confidence heal, strengthen and energize the body. In many ways, the brain doesn't distinguish between real and imaginary. If we visualize something happening then the brain can process it in some of the same ways as if it was actually happening. The brain is tricked into thinking that the fat is reducing and so it subtly alters our behaviour, cravings, motivation, as well as, perhaps, even how the body stores fat and where it is stored.

One of the bigger challenges in losing weight is getting

your mind aligned with your goals. More often, your mind is aligned with what you DON"T want – bad habits, laziness, avoiding exercise, and self-destructive actions of all kinds. Losing weight is hard under those conditions – if not completely impossible. One of the most effective techniques for bridging the gap between mind and body is visualization.

Visualization can help you lose weight in two basic ways: First, it can help you to overcome that inner voice. Second, visualization can be incredibly motivating. One of the major reasons why people give up on their healthy diet and exercise plan is because they just get bored with it. They get tired of eating the same old foods day after day, they get tired of doing the same workouts day after day, and they just lose interest. Visualization, along with your big WHY and SMART goal is a great antidote for low motivation. It's one of the best ways to renew your motivation each day and keep it going strong all the way to your goal.

So now you are asking the question, "What is Visualization?" Visualization is the process of seeing images in your mind. For example, if I asked you to think about an elephant, you'd probably see a quick mental image of an elephant. If I asked you to think about a red apple, you can see it mentally in your mind's eye. Most people don't have a problem seeing things mentally.

To use visualization for weight loss, you simply need to create little "mental pictures" about situations that you want to make true. It's important to note that visualization will be much more effective for you if you take the time to get very relaxed first. Feeling stressed or tired will make it harder for you to concentrate, and your visualization sessions will not be nearly as effective. Sit quietly and release tension from your mind and body. Breathe deeply and slowly, imagining that you are releasing tension and stress with every exhalation. When you feel relaxed and calm, then you can start with the following visualization technique.

Visualizing the End Result - The most common use for visualization is seeing the "end result" of the goal you are trying to accomplish. For weight loss purposes, you would focus on a mental image of yourself weighing your end goal weight and wearing the size and style of clothing you want to wear.
You might picture yourself in a certain setting that you've been looking forward to like a reunion of old friends, a wedding you have been invited to, a family gathering or just relaxing on the beach in swimwear.

You can also make the visualization more active by focusing on what you are doing at the time. Think of the answer you gave to your motivational questions. Perhaps you have a desire to be more active and healthier. So you might picture yourself jogging down the road with your head held high, oozing confidence with every step. Include as many details in this vision as you can. What clothes have you on? What way are you feeling? What do you look like? The more detailed you can make it the more powerful it can be. Try to make the vision so real and strong that you feel as if you are truly there, experiencing it right now. Stay with the vision for as long as you like – 10 minutes or so is great, but you can do it for longer if you wish.

Feeling the Reality of It - Imagine what it FEELS like to accomplish your goal both physically and emotionally. On the emotional side, perhaps you'd feel pleased, excited, proud of yourself, happy, and satisfied. On the physical side, you'd feel strong, empowered, slender, fit, and healthy. Focus on each of these for a few minutes, really tuning into the FEELINGS that they bring up within you. What would it feel like to be really fit and slim? What would it feel like to wear smaller size clothing and know you look great? What would it feel like to be so proud of yourself that you're ready to burst? FEEL it as if you are truly right there, living it now. It doesn't matter if you actually see any images or not, as long as you are tuning into the feelings that you want to experience when you've achieved your goal.

How Often to Visualize - To be effective, visualization really should be done at least once a day. You will probably be more committed if you set aside the same time to visualize each day. First thing in the morning is great as it sets a positive tone for the entire day. You can also try visualizing at night before bed, just try to make it the same time each day so you don't forget. Focus on feeling the satisfaction, pride, happiness, confidence, or whatever feelings would be associated with the outcome.

Be committed, be patient, and you'll reap the rewards!

DAY 3 - THE YO-YO CRAZE

"It is never too late to begin creating the bodies we want, instead of the ones we mistakenly assume we are stuck with."
Deepak Chopra

Remember the 80's Coca-Cola Spinners Craze! In the mid 1980's the UK and Ireland was gripped by Yo-Yo Fever and everywhere you looked, there they were. You couldn't open a newspaper or switch on a television with seeing Yo-Yos. Everyone knew about Yo-Yos and they didn't just go up and down. These Yo-Yos did all sorts of tricks. But ultimately no matter what angles and jumps they went through they ended up dangling at the end of the string

For most people that is the story of their diets, up, down, sideways, perhaps all sorts of fancy tips and tricks but ultimately they find themselves back to their original weight or worse even heavier. Has this been your experience? It certainly has been mine in the past. Now I am not beating you over the head for failing. Tiffany Wright, PhD, founder of Skinny Coach Solution tells us that "Every minute that you're at a healthy weight is beneficial for you. It's less stress on your heart and arteries, reduces your risk of disease, and increases your lifespan tremendously," she says. So well done, you were able to lose weight and losing weight benefited your health. Don't stop trying to lose the weight.

We gain weight until we come to a tipping point that makes us think "I need to lose some weight!" and then we do what everyone does, we go on a diet. There are plenty of diets out there to choose from but most follow a particular pattern, there is something, or a lot of things, that you have to abstain from. Eat no meat, eat only protein, cut out all grains, you know the story. How about 'The Mars Bar Diet," eat only Mars bars and in theory, you can lose weight. Follow these diet to the letter and you will lose weight, struggling along the way, fighting cravings night and day, to the point you can't take it anymore then you give in and binge. Once you stop the diet slowly or quickly the weight comes back.

What is going on, why can we not stay at the weight that we get to on our diet? A recently published report led by the World Obesity Federation has defined obesity as a "chronic disease". This is why we follow the yo-yo pattern. We work hard at the diet, lose some weight, but then our body starts to fight against us. Our body has a lot of tricks. As we lose weight our body tries to get us to put it back on again. It lowers our metabolism, increases our appetite and even our muscles become more efficient. When we have lost weight we can do the same amount of exercise and burn fewer calories.

With any treatable chronic disease, your doctor can prescribe medicine that helps or removes the symptoms. When the medication is stopped the symptoms come back and the risk is increased. It is the same with weight loss. Once you stop your diet, stop the exercise or medication the weight comes back. Obesity behaves like a chronic disease. It is not about shame or blame. The problem you are up against is the same as anyone who has a chronic disease.

The Holy Grail of weight loss, the key that will enable you to reach your goal is to get your body and mind working for you instead of working against you. This is not a daily struggle and battle of self-denial and cravings that need to be defeated. This is a journey to a good place, a better place, a place of health and energy. It is to be embarked on with enthusiasm and vigour. This is why our goals and picturing what it will be like at the end of the journey is so important.

"The idea of putting people on a "diet" is passé. It can

work against people if they think, 'I'm on a diet. When am I going to get off that diet?'" says Ann Cobau, a behavioural therapist with St. John Providence Weight Loss in southeast Michigan. What I am trying to do for you my friend is helping you change the way you think and behave in order to bring about long-term health and wellbeing.

As we continue to walk this journey together my aim is to help you keep changing your thinking as well as giving you lifestyle motivators that will increase and enhance the weight loss process.

If you are like me I need to ask you this question. "Did you do the pen and paper exercise that we outlined on day one?" I can't stress enough how foundational this is. Your WHY and SMART goal is what will carry you through to success. And here's a mega-super trick, if you really want to make it stick. Remember how teachers used to "punish" you by making you write sentences over and over again? It's actually a really good trick to make your subconscious aware of your goal. Grab a sheet of paper and write your goal down over and over again. Do this as often as you need to — without cramping your hand, of course! Don't think of it as punishment. Think of it as a way of communicating with your subconscious mind.

It is not inevitable that you will fail yet again. You can be the best possible you that you can be. Keep walking this journey and give yourself the strong, healthy body that you deserve.

And no, typing it up is not the same. Put pen to paper and really, really concentrate. Take your time and don't rush it. Make your brain pay attention to your goal — and your brain will then help you reach that goal. It'll seek out ways to help you because it knows your goal is important to you.

DAY 4 - UISCE BEATHA – THE WATER OF LIFE

"Water is the driving force of all nature."
Leonardo da Vinci

Uisce beatha - is the name for whiskey in Irish. The word "whiskey" is simply an anglicised version of this phrase. Uisce beatha, literally means "water of life", and was the name given by Irish monks of the early Middle Ages to distilled alcohol. It is basically a translation of the Latin aqua vitae which has also been used to describe the Fountain of Youth a spring that supposedly restores the youth of anyone who drinks or bathes in its waters. Tales of such a fountain have been recounted across the world for thousands of years, appearing in writings by Herodotus (5th century BC), the Alexander romance (3rd century AD), and the stories of Prester John (early Crusades, 11th/12th centuries AD). Stories of similar waters were also evidently prominent among the indigenous peoples of the Caribbean during the Age of Exploration (early 16th century), who spoke of the restorative powers of the water in the mythical land of Bimini.

Now have I got your interest, are you all excited? Do you think that my magic weight loss bullet is drinking lots of Irish whiskey or that I am going to reveal to you the secret location of the Fountain of Youth? Sorry to burst your fantasies but I am going to tell you that a key to losing weight and keeping it off is WATER.

Now water is something that thankfully we have plenty of in Ireland, sometimes far too much. And fresh spring water too. When I was a boy in the middle of our backyard there was a big deep well. The pure spring water was pumped up to a tap in the kitchen. Clean and cold and available whenever it was needed.

Water is one of the most important elements in the human body. It makes up about 60% of our bodies, more or less. Every single cell in your body needs water to function properly. The importance of water just can't be stressed enough. A person can go for weeks without food, but only a few days without water. Maintaining optimal hydration is essential for the body to function correctly, especially during exercise or in hot weather. Just to make it clear I am speaking about getting your fluids from water, not alcohol or excessive amounts of caffeine. Both of these contribute to increased urine production, making it more difficult for your body to retain fluids during rehydration. In most cases, tap water is as good if not better than bought or bottled water. You might want to think about purchasing a quality filter.

Because water is an appetite suppressant, drinking it before meals can make you feel fuller, therefore reducing the amount of food you eat. Health resource website WebMD states that drinking water before meals results in an average reduction in intake of 75 calories per meal. Drinking water before just one meal per day would cause you to ingest 27,000 fewer calories per year. Do the math: You'd lose about eight pounds per year just from drinking water! Now imagine if you drank it before each meal.

In one study of healthy men and women, published in The Journal of Endocrinology & Metabolism, drinking about 16 ounces of water temporarily spiked participants' metabolic rate by 30 percent. The researchers concluded that increasing water intake by 1.5 litres (about six eight-ounce glasses) per day would increase daily caloric burn by about 200 calories.

Higher fluid intake increases the amount of urine that passes through your kidneys, helping to flush toxins from them and supporting normal kidney functions. It also helps prevent the build-up of minerals which could turn into kidney stones. Optimal kidney function leaves the liver free to do its job as one of our primary fat-burning engines. If the kidneys are stressed, the liver has to pick up the slack. In other words – keep drinking to keep your liver happy!

So how much should you drink? Although everyone has different needs, sticking to the oft-recommended amount of eight 8-ounce glasses (64 ounces total) should be sufficient and can help boost weight loss for the average person or someone just looking to drop a few pounds. In general, you should let your thirst be your guide. If you're still thirsty after drinking 8 glasses throughout the day, make sure you adjust your intake accordingly. But if you're feeling quenched, be sure not to overdo it. A good key to preventing over hydration is to sip—not gulp—water throughout the day and to take in about half your body weight in ounces of water per day. For instance, a 140-pound woman should take in about 70 ounces of water per day. Add fresh fruits to your water and let the natural sweetness come through. Citrus peels, such as lemon and lime, can improve the taste. Don't be scared to mix in exotic fruits and fresh herbs like watermelon and mint or raspberry.

An old joke says you don't buy beer, you rent it, but the yellowish liquid in that ceramic bowl is no joke. Urine can offer tell-tale signs of what's happening inside the body it's departing. Straw-Coloured to Transparent-Yellow Pee is the normal urine colour of a healthy, well-hydrated body. It is the result of a pigment called urochrome and how diluted or concentrated the urine is. Pigments and other compounds in certain foods and medications can change your urine colour. The darker yellow or amber your urine, the more dehydrated you are, too clear and you might have to cut back a little on your water intake.

Drinking plenty of water every day is not only good for your overall wellbeing but also helps hydrate and tighten your skin after weight loss. Besides, it makes your skin smoother and radiant. Have it in mind that water plays important roles in nearly all body functions, and if many are compromised, the impact might reflect on your skin. Staying well-hydrated flushes out all the impurities which will leave you with a glow and a great complexion. You'll also notice your skin looking younger and healthier.

If you want to be healthier and lose more weight, drinking water is one of the easiest things you can do. Water and weight loss go hand in hand. You'll feel better than ever, you will look amazing and your metabolism will increase so weight loss and weight management won't be such a burden. It really is the stuff of life so get drinking.

DAY 5 - GOOD NIGHT

The Irish are renowned for late nights. There is nothing like a good night's craic (Fun) and late night ceilidh. Last century those late nights might have been accompanied by late morning as well. We live in a society where life is very fast paced. The normal tendency is that we stay up too late, then we wake up too early with the busy demands of the day upon us, and, increasingly, we find ourselves overweight.

One of the biggest mistakes that most people make [when trying to lose weight] is not sleeping enough. According to the National Sleep Foundation, your body repairs itself by releasing growth hormones while you sleep. Those hormones stimulate muscle and protein synthesis, as well as a fat breakdown process called lipolysis. Sleep is not a quick fix, but consistently having a quality night's sleep could be the secret ingredient for your weight-loss plan.

While there's plenty of data showing that poor sleep can lead to weight gain and possibly even obesity, some new research also shows that the opposite may also be true: that getting the right amount of good quality sleep may actually help you shed a few pounds. Matthew Walker, a professor of psychology and neuroscience at the University of California, says "Getting a full night of sleep is one of the most under-appreciated factors contributing to healthy weight maintenance," A 2013 study by University of Colorado researchers showed that losing a few hours of sleep a night for a few nights in a row can result in weight gain. *

A study of 1,024 volunteers that showed that when people didn't get enough sleep, their hormone levels became unbalanced. Their levels of the hormone leptin, which is responsible for feeling full, dropped, and the levels of the appetite-inducing hormone ghrelin went up. Researchers think sleep helps our bodies keep those hunger hormones in line, making sure that we feel hungry only when we should.

Sounds good but how can I accomplish it. I meet so many people who struggle with sleeping all night and certainly have had my share of restless nights, tossing and turning. The first tip ties in well with our overall weight loss theme. Don't eat before bed. Those late night searches of the fridge or cupboards looking for a little snack to tide you over need to end. If you want to improve your sleep this is a good rule to stick to. Detox expert, Dr Alejandro Junger advises you should keep a 12-hour fasting window at night. So, if you usually wake up at 7.30am, don't eat after 7.30pm the night before. He says, 'This is because your body won't slip into deep detox mode until about eight hours after your last meal and then it needs about four more hours of undisturbed sleep to do its job properly.' A study by the American Journal of Gastroenterology also found a significant link between late-night eating and acid reflux symptoms. So, it could not only harm your sleep but also make you ill in the long run. Avoiding caffeine later in the day can also definitely aid in a good night's sleep.

You probably already know this, but the light emitted from your phone, computer, and tablet promote wakefulness. The blue light produced by screens messes up your internal circadian clock by making your brain alert at a time when it should be asleep. Also, all of that stuff you are looking at — emails, news, and political rants — are not conducive to relaxation and sleep. In order to successfully drift off to dreamland, you might want to consider giving yourself a screen curfew. Since sleep is supposed to be relaxing and rejuvenating, consider activities before bed that promote this feeling. A bath, or reading a good book are both good ideas.

Turn out the lights—all of them. Forget a night light, a

bathroom light, or even a lighted alarm clock. Pitch black darkness is ideal for solid sleep, says research done by The Endocrine Society.

Having a consistent bedtime routine is also of real benefit. A warm drink, a good story, and a kiss goodnight aren't just a sleep recipe for Tots. Adults thrive on regular sleep routines as well, according to a study done by Brigham Young University. Setting and keeping, consistent times for going to bed and waking (even on weekends!) were the key to sleeping like a baby, the researchers found. (Bonus: It also helped the participants lose weight and body fat.) In addition, having a bedtime routine that includes things like reading a book, meditating, praying, and drinking herbal tea can help you relax into dreamland. Your body and mind will learn to recognize and anticipate these sleepy-time cues, leading to a smoother transition to good sleep. "Going to bed at the same time every night is important," says Dr Sujay Kansagra, director of Duke University's Pediatric Neurology Sleep Medicine Program. "It keeps your internal circadian rhythm happy and makes it easier to fall asleep." He suggests, however, that instead of stressing out about trying to achieve an unrealistic goal of a strict 10 p.m. bedtime, which you find a time that works best for your individual schedule and stick to it.

The National Sleep Foundation generally recommends that adults sleep for seven to nine hours every night, in order to wake up refreshed and alert for the day ahead. So when Mum used to chase us to bed encouraging us to get a good night's sleep maybe she knew as much or more than today's scientists. Go ahead try it, follow these tips and get yourself a good night's sleep.

"As a well-spent day brings happy sleep, so a life well spent brings happy death."
Leonardo da Vinci

* time.com/4757521/sleep-yourself-slim/

DAY 6 - THE TIMES THEY ARE A-CHANGING

When last did you have a long walk? What we would call a dander or might be properly called a stroll (which the Cambridge Dictionary defines as - to walk in a slow, relaxed manner, especially for pleasure.) Surgeon and obesity researcher Warren Peters draws a clear distinction between the way life used to be and our modern fast society (Yes even in Ireland it can be fast paced at times). We are basically the same people biologically but the environment in which we live has radically changed. My grandfather had a small farm in West Cork. I have early childhood memories of the Hay being cut with a scythe, turned in the sun with a pitchfork and then brought in from the fields in a donkey and cart. All by hand apart from the effort of the donkey which always had to be pulled and coerced anyway.

Consider this contrast.

How many calories would it take to get yourself a fast food meal from a drive-through restaurant? To keep the maths simple let's assume that your fast food meal amounted to about 2000 calories. With a few extras and going large I could easily have achieved that before I changed my thinking and lifestyle. Now in contrast, and I will use a classic Irish vegetable, that would be the equivalent of about 20 potatoes. Think of bringing those 20 potatoes to the table in the pre-machinery agriculture era (still with living memory of some of my much older friends.) The ground had to be dug and formed into drills, the seed potatoes had to be planted. As the plants grew, weeds would have to be pulled. Then the harvesting, the physical labour of digging the potatoes out of the ground, carrying them to the house, cleaning and preparing them. How did you cook them in the days before electricity? (Again some of my senior friends remember electricity coming to their rural areas.) Wood would have to have been chopped or at the very least coal carried in for the stove. I can't even begin to estimate how many calories in total would be used up in this whole process.

Back to the drive-through. You drive around the building and push a button to put your window down. That might take a couple of calories. You order your double, triple large meal and drive around another corner to the next window. Here it gets difficult for you have to reach out your arm twice, once to pay and once to pick up your order. With your meal safely in the car, there is one last task to be carried out. Push the button again to wind up the window and you are away. Obtaining your 2000 calorie drive-through meal has used up somewhere in the region or 10-20 calories at the very most. Do you see the problem here and some of the root of the modern obesity problem?

Now think about the types of food that we are buying and consuming compared to what our Grandparents bought and ate. In fact just over 30 years ago the bulk of money was spent on meat, fruit and vegetables. Real food. Food from the farm not from the factory. Today the vast majority of the shopping bill goes on highly processed foods. The modern food industry produces over 88,000 individual processed foods, 82 percent of which have added sugar. This has created a "system overload" in humans and sugar addiction. Many children today don't even know where real food comes from. Walk into any shop in the Western world and you are bombarded with all sorts of varieties of sugar-laden goodies. From sugary breakfast cereals to whatever we eat last thing at night. Is it any wonder that you need to make lifestyle choices that are counter to the environment all around us?

I have happy memories of family Christmas celebrations.

Of the many things that stand out two things always meant Christmas in Ireland. The first was a big tin of chocolate sweets. The second was the selection boxes or stockings full of yummy chocolate bars. Why do these two things stand out in my memory? Simply because they were not the norm. They were treats. The things that were unknown to my Grandparents, rare to my parents and treats to me in our childhoods are now common and plentiful.

In 1898 the first car came to Ireland. Medical practitioner Dr John Colohan imported an 1898 Benz Velo Comfortable to Dublin. My grandmother would have been 2 at the time. In just over a 100 years, cars that were unknown and then rare are again the normal mode of transport. After analysing national statistics between 1985 and 2007, researchers at the University of Illinois found that vehicle use correlated 99% with annual obesity rates. Not surprising is it as it stands to reason that the less you bike or walk, the more you drive. And the more you drive, the less exercise you get.

Then there is television. The first TV broadcasts were received in Ireland in 1949. It was 1962 before Ireland had its first public broadcasting station. A recent study published in The American Journal of Clinical Nutrition found that the more hours spent watching television, the more likely children were to be both fatter and less physically active. 89 children from Scotland between the ages of 2-6 years were recruited for a study, in which total energy expenditure and physical activity were measured. The parents were asked to fill out questionnaires detailing television viewing habits. The researchers found a significant association between the number of hours of television watched per day and body fat mass, with every extra hour/day spent watching television associated with a 2.2 pound increase in body fat.

We could keep going speaking of the multitude of environmental, social and technological changes that have taken place in living memory that have transformed our world. Many of these have had a negative effect on our body weight. Our challenge is to take a long hard look at our own lives and think "What can I change that might even in a little way combat or change these negative influences on my life?"

Can you think about buying food that comes from a farm, not a factory? Do you really need that sugar-filled goodie, or can it be kept for a treat at a special occasion or not at all? Do you really need to use the car for that short journey or could you possibly walk instead? Do you have to watch that TV program or could you go out and do some gardening?

Don't let yourself get swept along with the ever faster environmental changes all around us. Step to one side and think, "What can I do differently that will improve my health and help me to lose weight?"

DAY 7 - GET MOVING

My grandmother was a wonderful lady who lived into her 103rd year. When I was a boy I remember her walking several miles to visit us. I cut her grass and weeded her garden and she was always out supervising, poking at the weeds with her walking stick, keeping me right. Whether she knew it or not, her refusal to stop moving contributed to her health, mentally and physically. Following on from Day 6 we see the importance of being counter-cultural to our high tech environment and the need to get moving. Evelyn O'Neill, manager of outpatient exercise programs at the Harvard-affiliated Hebrew Rehabilitation Centre, sees the consequences of too much sitting every day. "Sitting is the new smoking in terms of health risks," she says. "Lack of movement is perhaps more to blame than anything for a host of health problems." Scientists are now linking a sedentary lifestyle (defined as sitting for twenty-three hours a week or more) with diabetes, high blood pressure, cancer, cardiac disease, and premature death. On the flip side, squeezing in extra movement during the day can have a big impact. For instance, simply standing more can help you lose weight and keep it off, according to a review published in the European Journal of Preventive Cardiology.

You were made to move and move often. "Walking is a man's best medicine", said Hippocrates over 2,000 years ago – and a growing body of scientific evidence suggests he wasn't wrong. This is where I suggest you start. No other exercise provides the same health benefits as walking does. Not running, cycling, lifting weights or anything else. Swimming comes close but is logistically harder to do. Walking is defined as "moving at a regular pace by lifting and setting down each foot in turn, never having both feet off the ground at once." It is suitable and safe for almost everyone – regardless of age, fitness level or ability. The statistics don't lie. The average person will burn around 300 calories an hour, so if you just walk for half an hour six days of the week without eating less you'll lose a pound – almost a stone over a year - and the faster you walk, the more calories you'll burn. Eat a bit less and up your walking and you'll lose even more. Brisk walking speeds up your metabolism – the rate at which you burn calories – not just while you walk but for several hours afterwards and you'll burn even more with intervals of high intensity walking.

Walking might seem unglamorous next to more calorie-intensive and sweat-buffed popular options like cycling and running, but it comes with several key advantages. Its low intensity, which means it's easy on the joints, helpful for promoting blood flow, and hard to mess up. And because it raises your heart-rate without sending it thudding through your chest, it's also more likely to relieve stress than cause it: In comparison, running sends forceful shocks through your lower limbs, promoting the production of the stress hormone cortisol. And you do not need any fancy gear or special training to do it. There's no mental preparation, no getting prepared the night before or monthly gym fees and it can be done almost anywhere at any time.

Walking is definitely the ideal way to lose weight and improve fitness. The hardest thing is taking the first step getting off the couch and beginning to move. Walking every day can build up your leg muscles, which may help you live longer. Researchers have found that loss of leg muscle strength and mass is associated with slower walking speeds among older adults. Slower speeds are linked to a lower 10-year survival rate for people after age 75. According to one study of 334,000 people by researchers at the University of Cambridge, just 20 minutes a day cuts your risk of premature death by almost a third. Yet Public Health England (PHE) has found that four in ten middle-aged adults – six million Britons – are failing to manage even one brisk 10-minute walk a month, increasing their risk of developing potentially fatal illnesses.

Did you know that there is a right way to walk? Your spine should be straight, with ears over shoulders, shoulders over hips, and hips over knees. Your arms should be bent at 90 degrees and swing back and forth (not across the body) from the shoulders. Your legs will naturally move in sync, so the faster you swing, the faster you'll walk. Your feet should land heel first with each step. You should then roll through the foot and push off with your toes. If you hear a slap-slap when your foot lands, you're landing too abruptly, rather than rolling smoothly. Go outdoors. Grass, sand, dirt, and roads are never completely level, so they work out muscles more effectively than a treadmill does. You also burn more calories when you contend with wind, which increases resistance as if you're walking up a small hill. Walking downhill is essential for building strength in the quadriceps and shins. Most people get sore after hiking on hills, not because of the climb but because their muscles aren't used to the descent. Set yourself a goal of a distance or number of steps. A time goal is too easy to fudge as you could be stopping to chat or stretch. The easiest suggestion is this: Walk as much as you can whenever you can. We know it has health benefits. So why not just do it?

This is a great point to end this chapter on. Walking makes you happy. It's true – exercise boosts your mood. Studies show that a brisk walk is just as effective as antidepressants in mild to moderate cases of depression, releasing feel-good endorphins while reducing stress and anxiety. So for positive mental health, walking's an absolute must. Are you inspired yet? A key part of my weight loss has been to get out there and to get moving by walking, walking, walking. No more excuses, get out there and move.

"Above all, do not lose your desire to walk. Every day, I walk myself into a state of well-being & walk away from every illness. I have walked myself into my best thoughts, and I know of no thought so burdensome that one cannot walk away from it. But by sitting still, & the more one sits still, the closer one comes to feeling ill. Thus if one just keeps on walking, everything will be all right."
— Søren Kierkegaard

DAY 8 – BACK TO NATURE

"In every walk with nature, one receives far more than he seeks."
John Muir

Put down your phone and experience the outdoors. Unplug and recharge in the wilderness. Long before smartphones and self-driving cars, Japan deemed "forest bathing" an essential part of its national health program. With forest bathing, the soaking isn't literal. Bathing takes on a new meaning—immersing yourself in the natural environment. There is something about getting into the midst of the ruggedness of nature that does the soul good. When we leave behind the crowd, the ease of the pavement/sidewalk, go where the way is tough and hard going. Revel in the sense of accomplishment of climbing a hill or mountain. Breathe the fresh air far from petrol fumes. Air quality is known to increase longevity and is better in areas with more dense vegetation. Feel the wind and sun on your face. Remind yourself that it is good to be alive. The human body thrives off of adversity and the beauty of nature. When we become disconnected from all hardships in the form of vigorous hikes, climbing mountains, the rain and cold and hot weather, we become weak and depressed. The nature that can only be reached and seen by using our own two feet acts as a natural medicine for the human soul.

In Ireland we don't often have to worry about too much sun, perhaps your climate is different and you know the precautions that you need to take to protect your skin. Using caution while out in the sun does not mean avoiding it all together. The sun provides the impetus for your body to produce vitamin D – which you need to absorb calcium. Many studies link weight gain definitively to vitamin D deficiency but only in the last couple of years have scientists discovered that your fat-burning metabolism is boosted with careful exposure to regular sunshine. That's right. In data published in The Journal of Investigative Dermatology, researchers discovered that subcutaneous fat burns faster with responsible exposure to the UV rays of the sun. In our modern world of the internet, streaming live television, and video games – is it any surprise that there appears to be an epidemic of vitamin D deficiency? Many people spend workdays indoors under fluorescent lights and in front of computers, then return home to bask in the glow of television screens. Switch off the gadgets, leave the comfy seat behind and get outside into the sunshine. It will make you feel wonderful inside and out.

If the main way your senses are stimulated is through watching TV or a screen of any sort you will become deadened to reality. Head outdoors and get yourself into nature. Wilderness, local woodland, Town Park or garden. Whatever is practical for you? Find a rock, log or bench and sit down. Quiet your mind, open your ears and eyes, and smell the flowers and foliage, become fully aware of your surroundings, soak up the scenery. Pick up a twig and feel its shape and the rough bark. Reconnect with nature. And don't just get out into the great outdoors when the sun is shining. In Ireland, we say that there is no such thing as bad weather for a walk just bad clothing choices. So dress appropriately for the weather and get out there.

After years of studies, medical professionals believe that strengthening your immune system will not only prevent weight gain but enhance weight loss. Staying indoors can have a negative impact on your immune health. The immune system works best when challenged regularly. That doesn't happen when we spend time indoors. What was once commonplace in society and for many of us growing up as we played outdoors, constant interaction with dirt, germs, and all sorts of organic matter teeming with bacteria, has now been replaced with an obsession to eliminate germs and provide an antiseptic environment. Immunologist Mary Ruebush, Ph.D. in her book "Why Dirt Is Good: 5 Ways to Make Germs Your Friends," says, "Don't be so quick to wash the dirt off your kids, or have them do it themselves, especially with anti-bacterial soap. You could be hindering the development of their immune systems!" so encountering a little dirt in the great outdoors might just help us boost our immune system and strengthen our body for weight loss.

Spending time in nature has been shown to lower stress levels. Office workers with window views are more satisfied and less stressed at work. Seattle-based environmental psychologist Judith Heerwagon says "Just looking at a garden or trees or going for a walk, even if it's in your own neighbourhood, reduces stress. I don't think anyone understands why, but there's something about being in a natural setting that shows clear evidence of stress reduction, including physiological evidence -- like lower heart rate." Bloodstream levels of the stress hormone cortisol are lowered after time spent outside. For a group of male students in China, those who spent their break from school hiking and camping returned with lower cortisol levels than those who spent time in the city. And these lower cortisol levels persisted for several days after their retreat to the wilderness. One reason Mother Nature may work as such a great stress-buster is through scent. The smell of many flowers, including jasmine, lilacs and roses, have been proven to decrease stress and increase relaxation. The scent of fresh pine has even been shown to lower depression and anxiety. Less stress equals more weight loss.

What has this got to do with weight loss, with reaching our goal? We not only want to lose weight, we want to feel fully alive. If depression and overeating go together then it stands to reason that when we feel good, when we feel alive, our very inner being will drive us to keep going in that direction. We will want to exercise more and we will want to eat the right nutrients to give us the energy and strength that we need. Spending the majority of our time in enclosed spaces such as cars, trains, shops, offices and houses is not who we were designed to be. So get out into the wide open spaces and live.

☐

DAY 9 - DO YOU HAVE AN ADDICTION?

I visited with an elderly uncle and aunt recently, 92 and 91 years of age. Now they have various age-related difficulties and are living life at a slower pace than they used to but both are doing remarkably well for their advanced years. The sobering thing in the conversation however that made me sit up and think was when they were telling me about their two sons my cousins. One has had complete Kidney failure and though he recently received a kidney transplant is struggling with health and the other recently had cancer. Now, this chapter is no reflection on their personal circumstances but it did lead me to think of the oft-quoted statistic that children born today will be the first generation to not outlive their parents?

Dr. Sreedhar Potarazu an acclaimed ophthalmologist and entrepreneur reminds us, "Twenty years ago, the incidents of obesity, alcohol, drugs, depression were not as prevalent. As a society, the future of our youth is truly at risk and many of these issues are interrelated. How we address them will determine whether our kids will really live longer than their parents." There is a multitude of reasons for the increased mortality rate among the younger generation. These factors apply to our western societies. Car accidents are a leading cause of death. We have a generation that is drowning in alcohol and drugs. Heart disease, some caused by smoking is on the increase. The impact of mental health issues has significant health consequences. What we want to consider in this chapter is the rising rates of obesity that has reached epidemic levels.

Many young people are now so grossly overweight they face premature death caused by a heart attack or stroke. The impending health disaster is blamed on the rise of aggressively-marketed, fat-laden fast food and couch potato lifestyles. One in ten children starting school in Britain is now regarded as alarmingly overweight, increasing to 15 per cent of school leavers. The main culprit – SUGAR. How much sugar do people in Britain consume? The National Diet And Nutrition Survey – based on self-reported consumption – is the nearest we can get to the truth. It gives the figure of total sugars: 96.5g per day – almost 23 teaspoons a day, or 160 a week.

According to the American Heart Association (AHA), the maximum amount of added sugars you should eat in a day are:

Men: 150 calories per day (37.5 grams or 9 teaspoons).
Women: 100 calories per day (25 grams or 6 teaspoons).

To put that into perspective, one 12oz can of coke contains 140 calories from sugar, while a regular sized snickers bar contains 120 calories from sugar.

So we need to ask the question, how did our food system get taken over by sugar? For the answer, we have to go back to the 1950s. As we prospered, it was relatively easy for the new industrial barons to figure out how to sell us more clothes, shoes and jewelry, for example. They could all be advertised as 'aspirational'. But one product proved resistant: food. Then the chemistry of processed food began to develop, with a growing understanding of how our palates and senses work. Manufacturers realized that by putting sugars directly into processed foods, they could manipulate the amount we ate and make our desire for sweetness override our 'full' button. Over decades, the tiny amounts of sugar in bread, savoury ready meals and sauces crept up – an indicator of our growing sweet tooth. How and where we eat has changed. When I was a child, I'd have three meals a day, with a few snacks. Now we eat throughout the day: at our desks, in the car, on the bus. We eat for fun. And so we end up eating when we are not hungry.

Scientists have found that sugar is addictive and stimulates the same pleasure centres of the brain as cocaine or heroin. Just like those hard-core drugs, getting off sugar leads to withdrawal and cravings, requiring an actual detox process to wean off. This may be why people say they can't resist the temptation to snack on junk food even when they desperately want to lose weight. The more they eat, the more they want, and it is the same mechanism as craving a drug.

Have you heard about the rats who found sugar or saccharin more tantalizing than cocaine? That's right, in a fascinating study, most of the rats studied — a whopping 94 percent — wanted sugar or saccharin, not cocaine. Dr. Serge Ahmed carried out research on "Food Addiction: The Obesity Epidemic Connection." He was researching the question, "Is Sugar as Addictive as Cocaine?" Ultimately, Serge and his research team discovered that intense sweetness "is much more rewarding and probably more addictive than intravenous cocaine." Serge concludes: "When society finally discovers that refined sugar is just another white powder, along with pure cocaine, it will change its mind and attitude toward refined food addiction."

Renowned addiction researcher Dr. Bartley Hoebel of Princeton University's Neuroscience Institute found that sugar can act on the brain in ways similar to drugs of abuse. Dr. Hoebel's rats even went into withdrawal symptoms. Their "teeth started chattering," Dr. Hoebel said. "They waved their heads back and forth. Their forepaws quivered. They acted anxious in a maze test. These are all signs of sugar withdrawal. So why am telling you all this? Because, if you have an overpowering sugar habit, I want you to know that this addictive feeling is not all in your head. You actually can get hooked. Even artificial sweeteners like aspartame cause withdrawal effects, so it's best not to use them as means to reduce sugar intake.

Megan Gilmore, a certified nutritionist consultant in Kansas City, Kansas says, "When you replace sugar with nourishing whole foods, your hormones will naturally regulate, sending signals to the brain when you've eaten enough." As a result, you'll lose weight without trying so hard—often within the first week. So if you really are determined to reach your goal, this is essential. Be ruthless with all added sugar, it has got to go. Ideally, we wouldn't eat refined sugar at all. Read labels – there is often more hidden added sugar than you'd think. Also, take fruit sugars into account when considering your overall consumption: a smoothie may have the same amount of sugar as three or four doughnuts.

> *"Sugar is 'the most dangerous drug of our time' and should come with smoking-style health warnings."*
> Paul van der Velpen, head of Amsterdam's health service.

DAY 10 - PASS THE SUGAR, PLEASE

If you are to lose weight sugar has got to go. How do you do that when your brain is crying out "I want sugar, I need sugar, get me sugar." Now you are not going to like me, you're maybe even going to close this book and find something more comforting to read. For that reason I want you to remember your WHY and SMART goal before you do that. To succeed sugar has to go. How do you break the addiction? The simple answer is going 'Cold Turkey.' What, is it not better to wean myself off the sugar? I will just take one chocolate bar a day this week and cut that down to half a bar next week. The problem is just having a little less sugar today perpetuates your addiction. The Brains reaction to sugar needs to be halted in its tracks.

You are going to have to manage the withdrawal symptoms that you will face when your body is not receiving copious amounts of sugar. Just as a drug addict faces withdrawal symptoms when they go 'Cold Turkey' you might face signs like lethargy, irritability, crankiness and tiredness. This is one of the reasons why people chuck their diet plan so quickly. They might actually be experiencing sugar withdrawal symptoms. The danger is that we misread this signs and think that it is our body saying that we are hungry. It is not hunger, it is our body adapting to going off sugar and off processed food that we are so dependent on and tend to overeat. The first three days without sugar are the hardest. It will level out on days four and five. Then from day six on things will begin to get better. Keep going, press on and things will get better, keep your goal in view at all times.

Then you have to deal with any cravings that you might still continue to have. Though you have kicked the physical addiction you still have an emotional attachment to sugary foods. Addiction is a very powerful form of learning. We have learned to associate different food triggers with the sugary foods that we eat. Now we have to learn to deal with these triggers and rewire our brain. Sound can be a trigger. Think of the sound of the ice cream van. You are sitting very contentedly then you hear the sound of the ice cream van and it sets your brain into overdrive, your reward system tingling and now you are thinking, "I would love an ice-cream." Another real trigger in our western world is fast food signs. The moment we see the signs advertising the well-known brands of fast food and surgery drinks, these logos become a trigger. They activate the brain reward system and virtually compel us to go and get food. You need to break the association. We will not even mention delicious smells in case you drop this book and run out to the shop. Sorry, the hard answer again is 'Cold Turkey.' The longer you can go without giving in to the siren call of the trigger, the easier it is going to get. So drive or walk right on by, do not give into the temptation of a quick sugar fix. The longer you can do that and the more often you can do that the less noticeable will be the pull of the triggers and easier it will be for you to keep on walking past them.

So what do you do if, or when being realistic, you relapse? I went to chop up some vegetables and my daughter had left a bar of white chocolate half eaten and the wrapper open on the worktop right beside the chopping board. It was almost as if she had given a lot of thought to 'how best can I put Dad under the most temptation.' My motivation was strong enough to close it over and put it away but that is not the way it would have been in the past. The 'just one little bit' would have soon have become a big bit or just the rest of the bar. The problem is that our environment is so full of triggers and easily available sugar fixes, it sets us up for a relapse. The important thing is not to beat ourselves up when we relapse. You simply need to set a goal of going longer the next time without a relapse. Remember this is not a battle of the will. It is breaking the thought and behaviour patterns that continually drive us toward sugar. When they are gone then the battle will be gone too. Knowing that you have done well to go so long without sugar and then setting a goal of doing better the next time can see you through your relapse.

The big red flag warning is this, don't do what I have so often done in the past. You give in, you relapse in whatever form that takes, then you say to yourself, 'well I have blown it now I might as well eat my fill and enjoy it and I will get back on my diet tomorrow.' Do not feed your addiction. Recognize that you have failed and plan to do better tomorrow and the next day keep going towards your goal. If you feed your addiction it will grow, if you starve it, it will diminish because you're not feeding it. If you continue to not feed it, it will fade away.

The last step you need to take to beat the sugar addiction is to develop a new way of eating. We need to have a plan for how we are going to cope when we find ourselves in a social or work situation and begin to crave that cake that is being passed around. Come up with a distraction plan to help until the craving passes. Tap your fingers, snap an elastic band or my forever favourite, go and get a glass of water to drink. I know it is not easy. Recently at a meeting at which a box of sweets was offered around a man said, 'you are not getting out of the room until you eat one.' I had to wait until he was at the bathroom and then make my escape. I am seriously considering self-diagnosing myself with a sugar allergy that makes me swell up so that I can tell people, 'well I will take it if you insist but I hope you are ready to rush me to the hospital.'

Learn to replace the junk and feed your brain with essential nutrients from natural sources. Instead of the sugar (dopamine) rushes from sugary foods the effect of healthy foods will leave you feeling full and fortified strengthening you in your recovery from sugar addiction.

"If you can quit for a day, you can quit for a lifetime."
— Benjamin Alire Sáenz

DAY 11 - WHICH DIET IS THE BEST?

It is the best diet in the world and it really works. It has been researched by the top government scientists and health experts of almost every country and they all agree. If you go to your doctors and you have an obesity problem he will pull the booklet off the shelf describing this diet and that will be your problem sorted. It is the, hold on a minute, it doesn't work like that, does it? Different health nutrition experts contradict themselves. The average person trying to lose weight tries four different new diets each year. 90% of dieters fail and 90% of dieters try to "eat less and move more" by adopting a variety of tactics.

My goal in writing this book is that you will be in the 10% that succeed. There is a very simple logical reason why diets don't work. Now, remember that we are trying to get our mind and our body to work for us not against us. We don't want weight loss to be a constant battle against cravings and temptations but instead a good and positive experience.

To help us understand this we need to define what we mean by diet. In the context that we are thinking of it means, "A special course of food to which a person restricts themselves to lose weight." We have already stated that you can lose weight on even the most bizarre types of diets. Ever hear of THE BEER AND SAUSAGE DIET. Evo Terra, 44, an online executive in Tempe, Arizona, dropped from 195 to 177 pounds in 30 days consuming an average of about 1,500 calories a day—

mostly from high-quality sausage and craft ale. So why am I saying then that diets don't work? Because they don't! You have been on a diet haven't you, in fact, more than one I am sure, but here you are reading this book because you are still struggling with weight issues.

95% of people who lose weight by dieting will regain it in 1-5 years. Since dieting, by definition, is a temporary food plan, it won't work in the long run. Moreover, the deprivation of restrictive diets may lead to a diet-overeat or diet-binge cycle. And since your body doesn't want you to starve, it responds to overly-restrictive diets by slowing your metabolism which of course makes it harder to lose weight.

Fad diets can be harmful. They may lack essential nutrients, for example. Moreover, they teach you nothing about healthy eating. Thus, when you've "completed" your fad diet, you simply boomerang back to the unhealthy eating patterns that caused your weight gain in the first place!

The main problem with most diets is that the body naturally works against them. Here in Ireland, a common expression is "I'm starving." My teenage son will come home from school, after having a healthy breakfast and a big lunch, come into the kitchen and announce, "I'm starving, what can I have to eat?" That is just the natural cry of a growing boy. His body needs plenty of fuel to do what it is doing, living an active lifestyle and growing. The problem with restrictive diets is that your body then begins to cry, "I'm starving, and I need to eat!" So it begins to crave food, all or any sort of food. The fattier the better. This leads to a battle between your willpower and your body. You are trying to say no, I am trying to be good, your body is shouting food, food I need food. There is a constant ongoing battle. It's like your brain just locks in on a craving and dominates your thoughts until you give in—and then you can't stop beating yourself up for going there. It's a vicious cycle that leads to unhealthy choices and even more mind turmoil over the guilt and shame.

The key that we are aiming for is our body and mind to be working together to promote your weight loss and overall health. That is why it is so important the body feels satisfied with what you are putting into it and not continually fighting looking for what it knows that you need to survive. Your mind needs to be convinced of your goal. It ought to be looking for ways to help you not hinder you. Read your goal aloud – picture yourself accomplishing that goal. Eating a donut instead of an apple may seem rewarding at the moment, but thinking of the goal that you are working towards will provide a healthier perspective.

Your battle often boils down to a simple question: Are you really hungry? Ask yourself if you would eat a whole plate of cauliflower instead of whatever it is that you are craving. If the answer is no, you're not really hungry. Then you need to figure out why you think you're hungry. It could be that you're experiencing an emotional stressor that's triggering your thoughts of food and your desire to eat. Perhaps you are tired, upset, depressed, lonely, and anxious, in pain? Are you just bored? Simply recognizing that you're experiencing an emotion lets you shut down that inner eat-junky-food-now voice.

One trick that might help is to make it part of your daily routine to write down and commit to all your meals and snacks for the whole day in advance. Once it's written down, there's no going back. That way you know exactly what you'll be eating and when. This helps you block out unwanted thoughts about eating.

It is also worth being aware that Obesity and overweight can be conditions that are caused by early life trauma. There is well-documented research on the obesity-trauma connection. In one study of 286 obese people, half had been sexually abused as children. In these cases, "...overeating and obesity weren't the central problems, but attempted solutions." For these people, therapy might be a necessity for healthy weight loss--it could help clients identify the feelings and situations behind emotional overeating and replace it with healthier self-care patterns. (A much larger study of over 17,000 people provided further documentation of the links between "adverse childhood experiences;" unhealthy behaviours like smoking, drinking, and overeating; and mental, emotional, and even medical disorders later in life.) Your fitness is 100% mental. Your body won't go, where your mind doesn't push it.

"Success is no accident. It is hard work, perseverance, learning, studying, sacrifice and most of all, love of what you are doing or learning to do."
                                        Pele

DAY 12 – EAT YOURSELF THIN

"If you want to lose weight you might have to eat more."

Ok, this is not a diet book but we have to talk about food. If I am going to tell you that not restricting your diet is the way to go then how are we to lose weight. Yes for most of us we have to cut back on the amount that we eat, and we have made it clear that we are to kick sugar off the list completely in whatever processed form it might come. It is the quality of the food that matters. Losing weight starts in the kitchen, and what you eat is far more important than how you exercise because weight loss is 70% what you eat and 30% exercise. You can exercise daily and not see the scale move if your diet is not correct.

If we stop eating or drastically cut back on the number of calories that we eat what can happen? It can lead to Muscle Cannibalization. Drastic calorie deficits can cause this as well as not eating enough protein. This is simply when your muscles are broken down by the body and used as fuel for other parts of your body. To prevent this from happening a dieter must eat enough calories and enough protein to prevent this from occurring. Dieters want extra energy to come from their fat reserves, not their muscles or they're defeating the purpose. So, make sure you are eating enough to support your bodily processes and the growth and activity of your muscles, but not too much that your body won't burn a small amount of its fat reserves each day to make up for the slight deficit you are in. So, focus on getting healthier by eating nutritious food, eating enough food, and being more physically fit.

We don't want to starve our body making it fight against us in its need for the right nutrients. We don't want to stop eating but we need to be eating the right foods. The best way is to skip the boxed, pre-made food. Instead, pick up fruits and veggies and lean protein from the butcher. You're are trying to only buy fresh food. From the farm, not the factory. Raw foods also have more nutrition, so a salad with raw spinach will have more fat burning properties than cooked spinach would, so whenever possible have foods raw.

So what have I been eating during this period of rapid weight loss? Now, remember I am no expert. I am just sharing what worked for me. Some of the many delicious foods I enjoyed eating include:

Whole Eggs. Once shunned for being high in cholesterol, whole eggs have been making a comeback. New studies show that they don't adversely affect blood cholesterol and don't cause heart attacks. What's more... they are among the best foods you can eat if you need to lose weight. They're high in protein, healthy fats, and can make you feel full with a very low amount of calories. Eggs are also incredibly nutrient dense and can help you get all the nutrients you need on a calorie restricted diet. Almost all the nutrients are found in the yolks.

Leafy Greens have several properties that make them perfect for a weight loss diet. They are low in both calories and carbohydrates but loaded with fibre. Eating leafy greens is a great way to increase the volume of your meals, without increasing the calories. They are also incredibly nutritious and very high in all sorts of vitamins, minerals and antioxidants.

Oily fish like salmon, mackerel, trout, sardines and herring are incredibly healthy. They are loaded with high quality protein, healthy fats and also contains all sorts of important nutrients. Fish, and seafood in general supplies a significant amount of iodine. This nutrient is necessary for proper function of the thyroid, which is important to keep the metabolism running optimally.

Cruciferous vegetables include broccoli, cauliflower, cabbage and Brussel sprouts. Like other vegetables, they are high in fibre and tend to be incredibly fulfilling. What's more... these types of veggies also tend to contain decent amounts of protein. They are also highly nutritious and contain cancer-fighting substances.

Beef and Chicken Breast. Meat is a weight loss-friendly food because it's high in protein. Protein is the most fulfilling nutrient, by far, and eating a high protein diet can make you burn up to 80 to 100 more calories per day. Studies have shown that increasing your protein intake to 25-30% of calories can cut cravings by 60%, reduce the desire for late-night snacking by half, and speed up our weight loss.

Nuts. Despite being high in fat, nuts are not inherently fattening. They're an excellent snack, containing balanced amounts of protein, fibre and healthy fats. Studies have shown that eating nuts can improve metabolic health. Population studies have also shown that people who eat nuts tend to be healthier, and leaner, than the people who don't. For me, my nut of choice has been Almonds. They have a well-deserved reputation as a health food and are high in beneficial nutrients like magnesium, vitamin E and copper.

Fruit. Most health experts agree that fruit is healthy. Numerous population studies have shown that people who eat the most fruit (and vegetables) tend to be healthier than people who don't. Even though they contain sugar, they have a low energy density and take a while to chew. Plus, the fibre helps prevent the sugar from being released too quickly into the bloodstream. Flavonoids are plant compounds found in fruit and vegetables including apples, berries, pears, strawberries and radishes. They have long been celebrated for their antioxidant effect, which is thought to help prevent cell damage. High levels of fibre found in apples have been linked to lower cholesterol and blood pressure and a reduced cancer risk. They are also a good source of magnesium, potassium and vitamin C.

During my 40 days, most days I had a big bowl of Greek yoghurt with lots of fruit and berries mixed in and crunchy linseed over the top. If we are eating daily a little of the right nutritious food then our body is satisfied and will not suffer from cravings, hunger pangs and spend all day thinking about food.

DAY 13 – GO WITH YOUR GUT

"The road to health is paved with good intestines!"
— Sherry A. Rogers

One decade, we're told to cut fat from our diets to lose weight. The next, we're told to count calories. Then it's all about ditching carbs. But could it be that we've had it wrong all along and the secret is actually already within us? More specifically, within our gut? Tim Spector, a professor of genetic epidemiology and author of The Diet Myth [Hachette], says yes. "The more diverse your gut microbes, the more likely you are to be healthy and lean, and the more sparse your microbes, the more likely you are to be overweight." Many a morning after eating a large spicy meal or just a feed of junk food I would complain the next day as my body was complaining, 'my tummy is rumbly this morning,' as I suffered the consequences of bad food choices.

Optimal gut health has become a prominent focus in 21st century health. Poor gut health has been linked to many health problems including obesity, diabetes, allergies, autoimmunity, depression, cancer, heart disease, fibromyalgia, eczema, and asthma. The links between chronic illness and an imbalanced microbiome (or gut bacteria) keep growing every day. Your gut is a huge chemical factory that helps to digest food, produce vitamins, regulate hormones, excrete toxins, produce healing compounds and keep your gut healthy. Your microbiome, the vast populations of bacteria that live on and in your body, deserve some attention—especially if you're trying to lose weight.

It is virtually save to say that all modern research suggests that healthy gut bacteria is crucial to maintaining normal weight and metabolism. The sad reality is that several features of the modern lifestyle directly contribute to unhealthy gut flora. The taking of drugs such as antibiotics and other medications like birth control and NSAIDs. Diets that are high in refined carbohydrates, sugar and processed foods. Diets low in fermentable fibres. Add to these chronic stress, lack of sleep and chronic infections that are all too common. All these contribute to gut imbalance. Back to our often repeated theme, modern society is hindering our ability to lose weight.

Unhealthy gut bacteria has been shown to produce food cravings: A study published in BioEssays suggests that some microbes may drive us to eat doughnuts or another tempting treat. These gut bugs send chemical messages to the brain that sway our appetite and mood perhaps making us feel anxious until we gobble a square of dark chocolate or a sticky cake.

We want our gut to be fighting for us not against us. Right now, as you're sitting there, there's a battle raging in your belly. It depends on whether the good bacteria in your gut or the bad triumph not just how well you will digest your dinner, respond to allergens and fend off disease but it also helps determine how much weight you're likely to gain, or lose. We need healthy guts working to our benefit. Intestinal health could be defined as the optimal digestion, absorption, and assimilation of food. To help you lose weight we need to take steps to restore your gut health. There are trillions of microbes in your belly that will if you feed them well help you fight flab and win.

The best way to grow a healthy inner garden and make your gut bugs happy begins with your diet. Basically, it all begins with probiotics and prebiotics, components of food believed to play an important role in improving gut health. Probiotics are a type of good bacteria, similar to the ones that already reside in your gut. Ingesting these organisms aids digestion and helps change and repopulate intestinal bacteria. Prebiotics are plant-fibre compounds, also found in food, that pass undigested through the upper part of the gastrointestinal tract and help stimulate the growth of good bacteria. When pre- and probiotics are combined, they become an intestinal power couple working with you for weight loss.

Fermented foods deliver probiotics directly to the gut. What about a pot of yogurt a day? Look for products that say "live and active cultures" on the label, and be careful when it comes to fruit-infused flavours: Some are loaded with sugar, which can feed bad bugs. For even more probiotics, try Greek yogurt (I will talk more about this later) or kefir, a tangy dairy drink that's packed with good bugs. A 2011 Harvard study found that yogurt was more strongly linked to weight loss than any other health food.

Fibre does more than fill you up: Research shows that foods that are high in fibre help promote the growth of friendly bacteria. Take a good probiotic supplement. This helps reduce gut inflammation while cultivating health and the growth of good bacteria. Add more coconut. Studies demonstrate anti-inflammatory and weight loss benefits from adding Medium Chain Triglyceride or MCT oils. Coconut oil and coconut butter contain these fabulous fat-burning MCTs.

What you don't eat is every bit as crucial as what you do add to your diet. Fatty and sugary foods not only tend to lack fibre which is the ideal food for the microbiome but can also cause bad bacteria to thrive. And let's face it: If you're filling up with that bag of potato crisps, chances are you're not munching on celery sticks, blueberries and other gut-friendly eats.

The above recommendations are not miracle cures. They are the actions that lead to normalized gut function and flora through improved diet, increased fibre intake, daily probiotic supplementation, the use of nutrients that repair the gut lining, and the reduction of bad bugs in the gut. The right fats, including omega 3s and extra-virgin olive oil combined with a whole, real food diet can actually repair your gut and even increase good bacteria.

Every day we live and every meal we eat we influence the great microbial organ inside us - for better or for worse. If you are still in any doubt about the role of your gut in a book about thinking and weight loss, ponder this quote of Giulia Enders, author of the book "Gut: The Inside Story of Our Body's Most Underrated Organ." Very bluntly she says, "We humans have known since time immemorial something that science is only now discovering: our gut feeling is responsible in no small measure for how we feel. We are "scared shitless" or we can be "shitting ourselves" with fear. If we don't manage to complete a job, we can't get our "ass in gear." We "swallow" our disappointment and need time to "digest" a defeat. A nasty comment leaves a "bad taste in our mouth." When we fall in love, we get "butterflies in our stomach." Our self is created in our head and our gut—no longer just in language, but increasingly also in the lab."

DAY 14 – TAKE TIME TO CHEW

Food was made to be eaten, not drunk. Juicing vegetables has become an all-out nutrition craze, claiming to "detox," "cleanse," or restore your body and digestive organs while claiming to give you all the same benefits of their whole food counterparts in a drinkable, on-the-go package. Juicing your veggies is not the same thing as chewing them. You lose nutrients in the juice form and are left feeling hungrier afterwards. Not to mention all the hard work involved. Who enjoys cleaning their juicer after use? There is no research to show that drinking juice, instead of chewing, will help your organs do their jobs better. In fact, our bodies were designed to chew (looking at you, teeth). We feel fuller and more satisfied with chewing than from drinking. How did people survive for years before juicers were invented? They took their time and chewed their food well.

The fruits and veggies used in your juice no longer have the same health benefits you get from chewing them. Mainly because juicing destroys the fibre: That's the stuff that fills you up, keeps you full, promotes gut health, helps regulate blood sugar, fights chronic illnesses (like cancer and diabetes), and helps you maintain a healthy weight. Also, some of the vitamins and minerals get destroyed too. So you are actually just left with the sugar. When you chew your food properly, your body releases digestive enzymes in the stomach that helps to break down food so that your body can convert it into energy. When food isn't digested properly, you could suffer from digestive issues such as indigestion, heartburn, constipation, headache and low energy.

Thinking About Losing Weight

Healthy digestion and nutrient absorption begin with the simple act of chewing your food. The physical process of chewing food in your mouth helps to break down larger particles of food into smaller particles. This helps to reduce stress on the oesophagus and helps the stomach metabolize your food. When you chew each mouthful properly, you also release a lot of saliva, which contains digestive enzymes. As you release these enzymes into the throat and stomach, you further improve the digestive process. Throughout the chewing process, the body undergoes several processes that trigger digestion. Digestion is one of the most energy-consuming processes of the body, so it's essential that you help your body along by doing your part!

How many times should you chew your food? The number of times you chew really depends on the type of food you consume. Soft fruits and vegetables will break down more easily than chicken or steak, so you will need to make sure you chew your food as thoroughly as possible. According to the experts at Ohio State University, you should chew softer foods 5-10 times, and more dense foods (meats/vegetables) up to 30 times before swallowing. You would benefit from chewing until your mouthful of food is liquefied and lost all of its texture, and finish swallowing completely before taking another bite of food. Wait to drink fluids until you've swallowed. The Times of India recently highlighted Horace Fletcher, a late-1800s health-food guru (also known as "The Great Masticator") who was famous for chewing each bite 100 times before swallowing (and to this, he attributed his good health, strength and endurance).

Chewing breaks your food down from large particles into smaller particles that are more easily digested. This also makes it easier for your intestines to absorb nutrients from the food particles as they pass through. The longer you chew, the more time it will take you to finish a meal, and research shows that eating slowly can help you to eat less and, ultimately, to avoid weight gain or even lose weight. For example, chewing your food twice as long as you normally would, will instantly help you control your portion sizes, which naturally decreases calorie consumption.

It's good for your teeth. The bones holding your teeth get a 'workout' when you chew, helping to keep them strong. The saliva produced while chewing is also beneficial, helping to clear food particles from your mouth and wash away bacteria so there may be less plaque build-up and tooth decay. When large particles of improperly chewed food enter your stomach, it may remain undigested when it enters your intestines. There, bacteria will begin to break it down, or in other words, it will start to putrefy, potentially leading to gas and bloating, diarrhoea, constipation, abdominal pain, cramping and other digestive problems. If you rush through your meal with hardly any chewing, you're also not really tasting or enjoying the food. When you take the time to properly chew your food, it forces you to slow down, savour each morsel and really enjoy all the flavours your food has to offer. It takes time (generally about 20 minutes) for your brain to signal to your stomach that you're full, and this may explain why one study found people reported feeling fuller when they ate slowly.

Remember when chewing it is essential you eat. Chewing without eating food can be counterproductive. When you chew gum, for instance, you send your body physical signals that food is about to enter your body. The enzymes and acids that are activated when you chew gum are therefore released, but without the food they're intended to digest. This can cause bloating, an overproduction of stomach acid, and can compromise your ability to produce sufficient digestive secretions when you actually do eat food.

The way you chew is unique to you and is probably

deeply ingrained by this point in your life. In other words, you'll likely need to make a conscious effort to change the way you chew, but the good news is you can start with your next meal. Consider the picture of the family sitting around the dinner table taking their time to talk through their day, eating home cooked nutritious food. No rush or hurry, and mother advising the child, "Keep your mouth closed and chew your food." Contrast that with, food on the go, fast food, convenience food mindlessly eaten as your zone out in front of the TV. The takeaway message from today is simple. Eat slowly. Whatever type of diet you have chosen. Take the time to chew your food thoroughly. Savour the flavour. Think about how each piece of food is nourishing and sustaining your body. Filling you up and meeting your bodily needs and satisfying your appetite.

> *"When walking, walk. When eating, eat."*
> Rashaski · Zen Proverb

DAY 15 – THE LONG NIGHT

"To lengthen thy life, lessen thy meals."
Benjamin Franklin

As a schoolboy I was skinny. Through my twenties, I carried hardly any weight at all. Then something happened when I hit my thirties. Life was rapidly changing, marriage, children and stress (must make it clear that the stress didn't come from the marriage and children but from work and life circumstances) and the weight piled on. As I took some time for reflection and self-examination I could give you many reasons why this happened. One, however, was very clear. Late night eating. Big social suppers, it is Ireland after all. Raiding the cupboards and fridge before going to bed. It all had taken its toll. Logic just dictated to me that the longer I allowed my digestive system to rest between my last meal of the evening and breaking that fast with my breakfast would be of benefit and help me lose weight. In fact, a whole science and industry have arisen around this known as Intermittent Fasting.

There are two popular methods of intermittent fasting. The 5:2 or Fast Diet. This was made popular by British journalist and Doctor Michael Mosley. It comprises of 5 days of normal healthy eating within your recommended intake of calories and 2 fasting days. On the two fasting days, you don't fast completely but you reduce your calorie intake to 500 calories for women and 600 calories for men. Then there is the 16/8 or Lean gains made popular by fitness expert Martin Berkhan. This method involves a 16-hour fasting window and an eight-hour feasting window. An example would be to stop eating at 7:00 p.m. and then fast until 11:00 a.m. the next day. During the feeding window, two to three meals are consumed, consisting of healthy, whole foods.

I have been consistently using the 16/8 or what I call 'The Long Night' to aid me in my weight loss goal. We have already considered the need to cut out late evening and night snacking and this is really just an extension of this. When you eat a meal, your body spends a few hours processing that food, burning what it can from what you just consumed. Because it has all of this readily-available, easy to burn energy (thanks to the food you ate), your body will choose to use that as energy rather than the fat you have stored. This is especially true if you just consumed carbohydrates/sugar, as your body prefers to burn sugar as energy before any other source. During the "fasted state" (the hours in which your body is not consuming or digesting any food) your body doesn't have a recently consumed meal to use as energy, so it is more likely to pull from the fat stored in your body as it's the only energy source readily available.

What are some of the benefits of intermittent fasting?

Keeping with the theme and goal of this book our first of course is weight loss. To help us understand this consider the following experiment that was carried out at Salk University. They put two groups of mice on different eating regiments for 100 days. Both groups ate a high-fat, high-calorie diet. The first group was allowed to eat whenever they wanted, grazing throughout the day and night. The other mice had access to food only for eight hours at night since mice are nocturnal. The results were astonishing. Despite consuming the same amount of calories every day, the mice that ate on a restricted eight hours were nearly 40 percent leaner and showed no signs of inflammation or liver disease and had healthy cholesterol and blood sugar levels. The group of mice that nibbled day and night became obese, developed high cholesterol, high blood sugar, fatty liver disease and metabolic problems. Our body is designed for overnight fasting. This was the norm until 50 years or so ago when we began to eat more and eat for longer periods of time. Much like our brain needs to rest at night evidence suggests that the stomach and the body's digestive system need to rest from processing incoming fuel as well.

Intermittent fasting puts our body into a clean-up mode called autophagy, which is literally translated as "cellular eating." When autophagy occurs, a bunch of little guys called lysosomes go around gobbling up damaged cells, damaged mitochondria, and cancerous cells. These lysosomes and mitochondria are good guys, giving us energy for vitality and cellular regeneration for a vibrant life.

It may improve memory and learning. According to a study by SM Raefsky, intermittent fasting increases neuroplasticity (brain flexibility) and the production of new neurons, which "enhance learning and memory." This study also mentions that it dials up antioxidant defences, autophagy and mitophagy (the clean-up of our cells and mitochondria), and DNA repair (which slows down ageing).

It improves immune function. In another study mice that had been intermittent fasting had a stronger immune response to Salmonella infection than those who hadn't. *

It lowers inflammation. One of the main causes of inflammation is an excess amount of free radicals within the body, which causes cellular damage. Throughout our daily processes of just living, mitochondria – which are the "batteries" in our cells that give us energy – get damaged. When mitochondria are damaged, they release free radicals which cause inflammation, age-related degeneration, as well as DNA damage. Intermittent fasting helps eliminate the free radicals.

It can help activate longevity genes. Michael Guo said of his research, "We found that intermittent fasting caused a slight increase to SIRT3, a well-known gene that promotes longevity and is involved in protective cell responses,"

I have added in some of the science behind the benefits to help encourage you to give it a try. The old saying goes, 'No gain without pain.' I want you to grasp that the gain, the weight loss and benefits to your overall health far outweigh any discomfort you may feel. When your mind is convinced that this is good and healthy then it is easier to make the decisions to say no when the eating temptation comes along. Through my 40 days, I have been pushing and pushing the fasted length and seeking to restrict my eating to as few as hours as possible. Go ahead try it, no evening eating and then push your breakfast back as far as you can.

> *"You can have results or excuses, but not both."*
> – Arnold Schwarzenegger

For further information –
(https://www.mommypotamus.com/intermittent-fasting/)
* (https://www.ncbi.nlm.nih.gov/pubmed/26798034)
Please keep in mind that this chapter as with all this book is for informational purposes only and is based on the opinion of the author. It is not medical advice and is not intended to be a substitute for professional medical advice, diagnosis, or treatment. As always, please use common sense and speak with your healthcare provider if you have a medical condition that might contraindicate intermittent fasting or any other lifestyle change.

DAY 16 – SKIP A DAY

"A diet changes the way you look. A fast changes the way you see."
Lisa Bevere

Get out the old skipping rope and get jumping. Skipping burns more than 10 calories a minute and is good for strengthening your shoulders, arms, legs and butt. If you did two 10-minute sessions of skipping a day that would burn off about 200 calories. Do it every day and it adds up to over 1,000 calories a week. I think I have inspired myself to try it out. What if you skipped a whole day? Think of the calories you would burn before you collapsed in a painful exhausted pile. There is an alternative that though not easy is not hard. Building on your intermittent fasting why not fast for a whole day? And by a day I mean from after dinner one evening until breakfast two days later which could be actually around 40 hours.

If the average man eats 2500 calories a day and I certainly was no average man often consuming much more than that. Then if for one day those calories are not eaten that would be the equivalent of you sweating and puffing as you attempted to skip with a jump rope for over four hours. There is an old Irish Proverb that says, "A fast is better than a bad meal." I suppose it all depends on how hungry you are. If you have eaten recently and don't need that meal to survive then it is definitely true.

For most of us we rarely and perhaps never have been in the situation where food is not readily available. This makes even the thought of not eating for a day totally unnatural. Taking steps towards it certainly, make it easier. Cutting out sugar should mean that you will not experience sugar cravings. Practising intermittent fasting means that your body is getting used to going extended periods of time without being continually gratified with food. Food is readily available but in a fast, you simply are choosing not to eat it.

Fasting for a day gives all the health benefits of intermittent fasting but in an increased way. Fasting lowers the insulin effect and insulin is the main driver of weight gain. Doctor Jason Fung also known as the Diet Doctor outlines these practical benefits of fasting.

Simplicity. Diet advice can be so complicated and contradictory that is bamboozles our brains. Fasting is so simple that it can be explained in two sentences. Eat nothing including sugars or sweeteners. Drink water, tea or coffee. Often the simpler a thing is the more effective it is.

Cheap. Feeding a family on a budget is a lot easier when you buy pasta and white bread. Organic and healthy foods can cost up to 10 times the price of less healthy alternatives. This does not mean you should be doomed to a lifetime of type 2 diabetes and disability. Fasting is free. Actually, it is not simply free, but it actually saves money because you do not need to buy any food.

Convenience. Eating a home cooked, prepared-from-scratch meal is terrific, but there are many people who simply do not have the time, ability or inclination to do so. Fasting saves time because there is no time spent buying food, preparing, cooking and cleaning up. It is a way to simplify your life. Where many diets complicate your life (eat this, but not that, and only a little of the other), fasting simplifies it. Save time and save money?

Power. Losing weight is hard. Everybody knows that. The most important question of any dietary intervention is this – will it work? Alone among dietary interventions, fasting is almost universally effective, since it is the fastest and most efficient way to lower insulin. It also contains almost unlimited power. What do I mean? Some diets have only one 'power' setting. If you follow the Mediterranean diet but fail to lose weight, then what? How do you become more 'Mediterranean'? It's impossible. There's only one power setting and it either works or it doesn't. Not so with fasting. You can simply continue fasting until the weight you desire is lost so there is unlimited power.

Flexibility. Fasting can be done at any time and in any place. If you do not feel well for any reason, you simply stop. It is entirely reversible within minutes. There is no set duration. You can fast for 16 hours or 16 days. There is no set schedule. You can fast a lot this week and none next week. It can change with your life's schedule.

Add to any diet. Here is the biggest advantage of all. Fasting can be added to any diet. That is because fasting is not something you do, but something you do not do. It is subtraction rather than addition. Simple. Saves money. Saves time. Flexible. Powerful. Available anytime, anywhere. What could be better than that?*

We have repeatedly stated that most of the battle with food is in our mind. If we have beaten the sugar cravings and learnt to extend our night time fasting periods then fasting for a day should not be beyond our ability. Hopefully, the above benefits will give you some additional motivation. We are so programmed with the need to eat that not eating can be a scary thought. Review your WHY and SMART goal. Fasting is of particular profit if you have stalled in your weight loss and can give it the impetus to get going again.

When you are fasting and you begin to feel the hunger pangs do something to distract yourself. You should be drinking plenty of water during a fast but have another glass or a herbal tea. Get moving and do some exercise or the opposite watch some television or a film. Don't focus on the foods that you are not having but on all the good that is coming your way. Do some visualization picturing how you will feel and look and the things that you will be able to do when you reach your weight goal.

One last motivator to keep you going. After you have been fasting, particularly if you have just been drinking

Thinking About Losing Weight

water, the first few mouthfuls of healthy food that you take and slowly chew and savour taste so so good. So why not skip a day and see the effect it has on your body.

"Fasting empties the stomach and the mind; freeing up space to refuel our bodies with the Bread of Life."
Allene vanOirschot

Do not go on a fast without advice from your Doctor.
* (For more information on these benefits go to www.dietdoctor.com/7-benefits-of-fasting

DAY 17 - STRESSED OUT

Eating too much and lack of exercise are the two main primary reasons for being overweight. Another contributing factor that we can't ignore is high cortisol which is mostly derived from chronic stress. What is cortisol and what does it have to do with weight loss? Cortisol is a form of hormone from the steroid family called Glucocorticoids. It gets triggered and increases when your body is feeling a little or more than a little stressed. Cortisol controls your flight or fight response. It is increased by physical stress but also by emotional stress. So if there is something that is causing you to freak out it is pumping your cortisol levels through the roof.

When your cortisol levels increase your body wants to get you out of that stressful mode and get you to be more relaxed. Your body is going to use a lot of energy to try and calm itself down and for this it needs glucose and glycogen. So what your body does is increase its cravings for bad foods. It needs glucose so it wants you to eat sugary foods. Your body is going to want that sugar and ask you for it.

Also raised cortisol levels are going to increase visceral

abdominal fat disposition, otherwise known as belly fat. This is that fat that is all around your organs and causes diseases. You really, really don't want that. As well as the cortisol, stress itself has been associated with overeating, which of course also results in fat gain.

What leads to this physical stress? Things like not enough sleep and too much caffeine. Doctors suggest that you limit yourself to about three cups of coffee a day or less. Not giving your body the proper nutrients that it needs can also lead to it feeling stressed. Stress leads to high cortisol. High cortisol will cause your body to demand glucose. High cortisol levels also can lead to muscle depletion. Your muscles have glucose in them and your body can pull this out to use. This is why you see people who are really stressed out sometimes getting skinny but not in a good way as their muscles are wasting away. Less muscle reduces your metabolic rate and can lead to weight gain. High cortisol can reduce your pituitary function which leads to brain fog, a drain in your energy and more stress.

Here are a couple of tips for helping you reduce your stress levels. Think back to a moment in time when you were happy and carefree. As you revisit that happy memory try to identify what sensations it evokes. It might be a sight, a sound, a smell touch or taste. When you've connected with this good feeling, close your eyes and rub your index finger and thumb together at the same time. Repeat this many times and each time make the feeling stronger. Make the sounds louder, the sight sharper and brighter and the smell more pronounced. Now focus on something unpleasant and then try rubbing your finger and thumb together and see whether you can bring back that positive feeling instead. What you have created is a triggered response. When you feel yourself getting stressed begin to rub your finger and thumb together. Your taking control of your thoughts, your taking control of your body, your taking control of your stress levels which takes control of your cortisol.

If you are feeling stressed physically the most important thing you can do is breathe. You have to bring oxygen into your body. When you are physically stressed, your body tenses up and you find yourself short of breath depleting your body of oxygen sources, this triggers your cortisol levels to go up to get you more glycogen to give you more energy. So breathe. We will look more at breathing in a later chapter.

Ireland used to be known as the as the land of Saints and Scholars and spirituality plays a big part of our heritage. Spirituality and faith have been proven to reduce stress levels. It was Jesus who said, "Come to me, all you who are weary and burdened, and I will give you rest. Take my yoke upon you and learn from me, for I am gentle and humble in heart, and you will find rest for your souls. For my yoke is easy and my burden is light," Gospel of Matthew 11:28-30. Prayer, meditation and similar practices have been associated with lower cortisol and other stress hormones (Koenig, McCullough 2001)

The ultimate Irish answer to any stressful situation has always been, 'sit down and I will make you a cup of tea.' Black and green teas are affordable and easy ways to reduce and regulate cortisol levels. In a randomised double-blind trial meant to show the effects of black tea consumption over a period of 6 weeks, results showed a reduction of cortisol levels as well as an increase in relaxation. (Steptoe A. et al., 2006). But hydration is also essential in maintaining good cortisol levels. A study performed on athletes exercising at different intensity levels suggests that dehydration leads to increased cortisol levels. So in order to keep stress hormone imbalances at bay, proper hydration is a must. (Maresh CM. et al., 2006) When you are feeling stressed put the kettle on and make yourself a cup of tea.

Here is an even better idea. The simple act of kissing can have a positive effect on one's cortisol levels. Through the use of blood work and an MRI machine researchers showed that kissing helps release oxytocin which in turn plays a role in reducing cortisol levels in healthy adults. (de Boer et al., 2012). Reducing cortisol can also be as simple as having someone to hug. A 2013 study tested the reaction between cortisol levels and interpersonal communication expressed through a hug. The results showed that the group that was allowed to use hugs to express themselves had significantly lower cortisol that the group who could only use words to communicate. (Hidenobu Sumioka et al, 2013)

If none of these are working, or there is nobody around to hug have you ever considered getting a pet? Playing with or petting an animal can increase levels of the stress-reducing hormone oxytocin and decrease the production of the stress hormone cortisol. In a 2001 study, researchers found that pet-owning patients with high blood pressure could keep their blood pressure lower during times of mental stress than patients without pets. Pets don't judge us; they just love us. Having a furry best friend can reduce stress in your life and bring you support when times get tough.

"He is richest who is content with the least, for content is the wealth of nature."
—Socrates

DAY 18 - TRICKS OF THE MIND

You have been trying really hard to eat less, stop overeating or to stop your snacking habits, but nothing seems to work? Remember we are looking for our body and mind to work with us not to be fighting against us. It is possible to learn to trick your brain into helping you instead of hindering you. Your mind can help you naturally to stop overeating without you even realising it.

Downsize your plate, downsize your portion. Research has shown that if you use a larger plate the tendency is to consume more food. If you use a smaller plate your eyes trick your mind into believing that you are eating more even though you are eating much less. In one experiment, conducted by Brian Wansink from Cornell University and Koert van Ittersum from the Georgia Institute of Technology, it was discovered that a shift from 12–inch plates to 10–inch plates resulted in a 22% decrease in calories. Assuming the average dinner is 800 calories, this simple change would result in an estimated weight loss of more than 10 pounds over the course of one year. Smaller plates cause us to eat less thanks to a powerful optical illusion known as the Delboeuf Illusion. The illusion works because we think things are smaller when we compare them to things that are larger. You can safely and happily eat a full plate of food and still lose weight, just start with a smaller plate.

Contrast the colour of your plate to your food serving. Researchers have discovered that when the colour of a participant's plate matched the colour of their food, they served themselves almost 30% more. In other words, if you ate pasta with red tomato sauce on a dark red plate, you ate almost 30% more than you would if you had used a white plate. The same was true for eating pasta with a white Alfredo sauce on a white plate compared to a dark red plate. When the colour of your food blends in with the colour of your plate, then the amount of food doesn't appear to be as large. The result is that you will end up scooping more food onto the plate. The higher contrast in plate colour to food colour will automatically prevent you from throwing an extra scoop onto the plate. Typically, this isn't something you will think about, your mind will just realize that you don't need another serving. You don't have to rely on motivation because the colour of the plate is helping your mind make the decision for you.

Drink tall and lose weight. Anything that is not water drink from a tall thin glass. Tall skinny glasses appear to hold much more than short glasses. Your brain will be tricked into thinking that you are actually drinking more from tall glasses than in comparison to short glasses.

Leave behind evidence of the food you have consumed. This is interesting particularly in the light of how processed and prepared our food can be. Picture two plates. One is completely empty almost as we would say in Ireland, licked clean. The other has some potato skins, chicken bones and the stalk of some broccoli on it, left after you have consumed a hearty healthy meal. Research says that when you give yourself visual clues to what you have eaten you consume 28% less food. The mind looks at the empty plate and forgets how much you have eaten and wants more, but it looks at the plate with the visual evidence and remembers how much it has eaten and is, therefore, more likely to be satisfied. Leave evidence behind of what you have eaten.

Take time to really appreciate your food. This goes along with our chapter on chewing. Look at your food, smell your food, taste your food, and really enjoy the texture of your food. This means that you should not eat in front of the TV or computer, do not eat while reading, basically do not eat when you are distracted. If you eat while you are distracted you forget what you have eaten. Scientists found that people who eat in front of the TV consumed 288 more calories than those who didn't.

Keep your food out of sight and out of mind. Research has shown that we tend to overeat if we can see the food and it is within our reach. This is particularly true of the temptation to snack while at your desk. Keep your environment clear of any food as much as you possibly can. The further away your food is the less likely you are to go and get it. Don't keep your snacks in a see-through container that you see every time you pass it.

Avoid food shopping when you are hungry. When you are hungry everything looks delicious in the shop and you just want to grab everything you see. Do you food shopping if possible after a meal when you are feeling full. This allows your mind to think about the foods that are necessary and good for you. Need not greed.

Have a starter before your main meal. If you fill up first on soups and salads it has been proven that you will eat fewer calories later.

The last trick, and if you are going to ignore all the others please give this one a go, eat with your non-dominant hand. That means if you are right-handed and using a spoon to eat out of a bowl, put the spoon in your left hand. Eating with your non-dominant hand causes you to eat, on average, 30% less, by preventing 'mindless' eating. Eating with your non-dominant hand forces you to think about what you are doing, to look at your food in the bowl. It slows the whole process down and really does lead to you eating less. The same goes if you are snacking nuts from a bowl, try using your non-dominant hand to reach out and take them.

Ok in and of themselves these tips are not going to lead to the rapid weight loss we are seeking to achieve but adding it all together they might be something in the above that will just give you a slight advantage and help you get over the goal line.

> "Slow but steady wins the race."
> – Aesop

DAY 19 – TECHNOLOGY AND WEIGHT LOSS

2018 began for me with a brand new resolution. I had often heard the mantra of walking 10,000 steps a day to lose weight. 10,000 steps came as a result of a marketing campaign in Japan in 1964. It was the run-up to the Tokyo Olympics and a company came up with a device called a Manpo-Kei. In Japanese "man" means 10,000, "po" means steps and "kei" means meter. The device was an early pedometer, literally, a 10,000 steps meter. It was obviously a super market success as it is still used as a benchmark today. Fired with enthusiasm for a New Year I bought myself a watch fitness tracker. It measures steps and heartbeat and links to my smartphone via Bluetooth. As I like to push boundaries I set myself a big goal of 20,000 steps a day. The amazing thing is that I actually managed to achieve this for the first five days. I had not thought this through properly. 20,000 steps are roughly 10 miles. Walking at a fast pace of 3.5 miles an hour meant that it took nearly 3 hours to achieve my goal. Add to this Irish winter weather which at that time was sub-zero temperatures and driving rain. Even the dog was beginning to run for cover when I shouted walkies.

It was too much at the wrong time of year and like all unrealistic goals, it and the watch was set to one side. I dug it out and dusted it down for my 40lbs in 40 days challenge. Remembering my mistake from earlier in the year I set a high but achievable goal of 16,000 steps a day. Better weather means early morning and late evening walks are very enjoyable. I redid my profile on the app and it gave me quite the kick in the backside. When I entered my weight the app gave me this stark statistic – "You are lighter than 3% of people compared with the same height users from the same area." Now I knew I was carrying a little extra weight but this app was telling me that I was classed as obese stage 1 and actually heavier than 96% of people in my area for my height. It was as if it was telling me, "Hey James you are the fattest person around." This was fuel to my WHY and added motivation that this time I was going to make a major difference to my weight and appearance.

Smartwatches and fitness trackers are commonplace today and vary massively in price. Mine is from the cheaper end of the range but has served my purpose well. The big benefit is in our often repeated theme, it helps to get you moving. Movement improves your insulin sensitivity - a measure of how effective your body is at processing excess glucose. Setting a goal on your device motivates you to get up and get going not just now and again but every day. Lots of wearables have inactivity monitors that you get set to vibrate if you have been inactive for a set period of time. These simply remind you to get up and move if you have been sitting at your desk or on the couch for too long.

Lots of research casts doubt on if wearing a fitness tracker helps you lose weight or not. For me the motivation it created every day to reach my goals was vital. In many ways, it was like my accountability partner helping to keep me on track. It helped to created lasting activity habits. I knew that I had to get moving early in the day in order not to leave too much to be walked towards the end.

It made my daily goals measurable. I wasn't saying I am going to walk more every day, but every day I will walk at least 16,000 steps and it told me when I achieved that goal. This meant that some evenings I had to get up and go for a long walk to make sure I reached the goal for that day.

Another fairly useful function that most fitness devices come fitted with is the sleep tracker. We have discussed the need for a good night's sleep if we are to lose weight. The problem is it is hard to tell if we are sleeping well or tossing and turning in fitful sleep all night. My tracker recorded the amount of time that I was asleep but also told me what type of sleep I had giving the percentage of deep sleep vs. light sleep and the times that I was awake. If you're tired this can make you more stressed then willpower is likely to go out of the window. That can be the difference between picking up some fast food or grilling some chicken breast at home instead.

As well as step counting and sleep monitoring there are plenty of apps for your smartphone designed to make calorie counting and nutritional tracking easier. Most trackers can be hooked up to Google Fit or Apple Health. MyFitnessPal always tends to top the charts. With its huge community of more than 80 million users, exhaustive food database and easy-to-use tracking features, it's no surprise that it's one of the top-performing apps. You might find an app like this helpful if not time consuming. But remember this is a 40 day challenge and once you have implemented a healthier lifestyle and it has become your habit rather than an exception then you can just keep walking that healthy way.

I used a simple app called "Monitor Your Weight." You added your current weight and your target weight and date to achieve it. Then every day of my 40 days I entered my weight for that day. On the home page, it gives a neat little graphic of progress vs. time so that at a glance you can see where you are in relation to your end goal. It also tells you your current BMI, how much you have lost and how much you still have to lose alongside your average daily loss and average weekly loss. I found that this helped and motivated me to keep pushing on every day to move towards my end goal.

I am glad to report that at the end of my 40 days my app was now telling me that I am lighter than 35% of people compared with the same height users from the same area. That fact certainly helps me stand taller and walk prouder.

"Success is the sum of small efforts - repeated day in and day

out." Robert Collier

DAY 20 – 4 STEPS TO CONFIDENCE

"The greater danger for most of us lies not in setting our aim too high and falling short; but in setting our aim too low, and achieving our mark."
Michelangelo Artist and Architect

Can you picture yourself, walking into a room of people, you have achieved your goal weight, you are tanned, fit and feeling good. Instead of shying away into a corner you are exuding confidence. I obviously don't know you personally, I don't know your character traits or if you are a confident person. But one thing I do know is that by losing that excess weight and reaching your goal weight it will boost your confidence.

If you are using this book as I did for a motivator and friendly helper as you walk through 40 days of weight loss tomorrow is a big day. When you weigh yourself tomorrow morning you will be at the halfway mark of your journey and hopefully, at the half weigh point of your weight loss. Congratulations. Keep going, keep visualising the new you that you are working towards. I want to share with you today the 4 C's Formula to build confidence created by Dan Sullivan.

The reality of this cycle, which applies to anything from personal exercise to business creation, first occurred to Dan when he was drafted into the Army in 1965. While in boot camp, his platoon was learning how to safely throw grenades — when asked by the drill sergeant who was scared, Dan was the only one of 50 to actually raise his hand. The sergeant then said, 'Sullivan is the only person here I trust because he's actually telling the truth — the people who are scared and don't say it, are a bigger worry to me than the people that actually admit it.' Later, after Dan had successfully thrown his live grenade, the sergeant commented, 'I want to tell you the difference between fear and courage: Fear is wetting your pants. Courage is doing what you're supposed to do with wet pants.'

I know you are excited about your weight loss and the breakthrough that you are almost halfway towards. Confidence is the reward for getting to your goal.

Here are the four steps:

Commitment – This is the first and most important step in your weight loss journey. If you are still thinking it would be nice to lose a little weight then you will struggle. That is why setting your goal was so vital. It is a definite commitment not just a vague hope. Losing weight is not easy and so many temptations and obstacles come across your path. Without steely, hard commitment the path will be fraught with dangers. This might be a good time to write out your smart goal and why again and recommit in your mind to achieving it. Read it out loud and then say something like "I am committed to achieving my goal. I am worth it." Without a clear commitment to achieve realistic goals you can't advance to the second step…

Courage - It's the courage part that feels really awkward because you have no proof that what you've committed to will work out. So you stop yourself before you even start because you're scared. Most people admire courage in others but don't like the experience themselves. Courage is when you say to your partner, children or work colleagues, I am going to lose (your goal) weight, fearing their reaction but you do it anyway. Courage = stepping outside of your comfort zone. Speaking up when you are offered something that you know will be detrimental to you attaining your goal, perhaps risking giving offence. As I write this I know that tonight I will be visiting some friends, a group that gets together from time to time. One of the key features of this evening is delicious food and lots of it. If you have ever seen the Irish comedy, 'Father Ted,' believe me that is what I will be encountering tonight. As the food is offered it will be accompanied with a chorus of, "you will, you will, you will," followed by "Ah go on, go on, go on." (Google 'Mrs Doyle Best Bits - Father Ted Compilation' if this makes no sense to you). I will have to risk offending when I explain that I no longer eat in the evening. It might be uncomfortable at the start but I know you have the courage to move through fear and demonstrate to yourself that you have got what it takes to succeed.

Capability – When you enthusiastically go through the uncomfortable courage stage, you quickly start to see a new capability emerging. You tried to lose weight in the past and failed but that was the past. Building up courage allows you to create the capabilities to succeed. You already have many capabilities. These capabilities increase as you read this book and other resources that equip and enable you towards your goal. This developing capability leads to the final stage of the four-step process,

Confidence - Don't expect to find the confidence right from the start. That's not the way it works. Confidence is the end product. Confidence is the resulting emotion that comes from being successful and overcoming your obstacles. Confidence embraces the ultimate skills you attained and personal improvements made. When you see that goal weight popping up on your scales the boost that will give to your confidence is enormous. Confidence is the natural result of what you have achieved. So the next time the fear creeps up, recognize it for what it really is… a gateway to confidence.

At this halfway mark it doesn't matter if you are bang on target or away behind, renew your commitment, take courage, increase your capabilities and press on towards confidence.

"Most people won't take action on a project or goal until they feel capable and confident about it, but those are stages three and four of the process. You can't have confidence until you have created a new capability, and you can't acquire a new capability until you have first made the commitment and then gone through a period of courage."
Dan Sullivan

DAY 21 – HALFWAY MARK

Congratulations! You are half way through your 40 days, that means that if you are following a rapid weight loss diet (Hopefully one full of the most nutritious food) and have been following the hints, helps and hacks in this book that you should be halfway to your goal.

Don't panic if you are behind. If your goal is to lose 20lbs in the 40 days and today you find that you have just lost 7lbs, brilliant. That is 7lbs you would not have lost if you had not started this process. Keep that rate up and you will have lost 14lbs by the end of the 40 days and then you can just keep going to you hit your goal.

The halfway mark can be a dangerous place. Everyone knows that fresh starts are great for motivation. Think of the crowds of newcomers signing up at the local gym every January or the rush of enthusiasm you feel when beginning a new project. Endings offer a similar excitement. When you're concluding a fundraising project or sales goal, you're likely to feel driven to reach the finish line. But what can you say for the middle of a project?

Motivation can be U-shaped, starting high, falling to a low point about halfway through and then beginning to rise again as we approach the goal we are aiming for. It's this midway low point that can be deadly to our dreams. The worst thing you can do is give in to the loud call of wrong foods and slip back into old eating behaviours and habits. Knowing that you are in this motivational valley of death, halfway to your goal, is half the battle. Look back at what you have already achieved and look forward with enthusiasm when you consider what it will be like when you have accomplished your goal.

The main thing is don't give up. As Winston Churchill is reputed to have said, "Never, never, never give up." Don't let this year be another year of good intentions with unaccomplished goals. The very fact that you have and are trying to lose weight and create a better you is extremely positive. Re-engage with your goal. Think of your original excitement as you thought of what it would be like when you reach your goal weight. The long-term gain of being a thinner, fitter you far out ways any short-term pain. Remember how important your goal weight is not only to you but also to your loved ones as well.

In the second half of the book, the chapters are going to be half the size of the first. What I am suggesting you do is that alongside each new chapter you go back and read one of the chapters from the first half. I know how easy it is to scan a chapter and not fully take in its contents. For you to take the best benefit it will be good for you to reinforce in your mind the teaching you have already received and seek to put it into practice.

"Winners never quit, and quitters never win."
—Vince Lombardi

DAY 22 – BREATHE

My friend's elderly father had just died minutes before I arrived at their house. He invited me to come into the bedroom to view his father's remains (don't worry it's an Irish thing.) There his father lay on the bed, but it wasn't his father. I speak respectfully but it was just a crumpled hardly recognisable shell. The breath had gone from his body and with the breath life. The book of beginnings puts it like this, "God formed Man out of dirt from the ground and blew into his nostrils the breath of life. The Man came alive—a living soul!" Breath equals life and when the breath goes life goes with it.

Breathing is something that we do automatically but just as we can have a poor quality of life we can have a poor quality of breath. We need to learn to breathe. What a beautiful thing it is to stand on a mountaintop where the air is pure and breathe in a deep lungful of quality air. But what has this got to do with losing weight?

Rather than changing your diet or getting fit, Jill Johnson's weight loss theory called Oxycise is based on a simple physiological fact working on the principles of aerobics - raising oxygen intake through sport. 'Fat is made up of oxygen, carbon and hydrogen,' she explains. 'When the oxygen we breathe reaches these fat molecules, it breaks them down into carbon dioxide and water.' 'The blood then picks up the carbon dioxide - a waste product of our bodies - and returns it to the lungs to be exhaled.

Therefore the more oxygen our bodies use, the more fat we will burn.' There is some validity to what Oxycise offers. Whenever the body is breathing in the manner laid out with Oxycise, there will be tightening of the muscles and an improved flow of oxygen as a result. This, in turn, can help to burn calories, which means some weight loss is possible. According to the principles of Oxycise, when we inhale and exhale deeply, the muscles in our body tighten because powerful breathing forces us to use our diaphragm.

This action of deep breathing naturally makes our muscles contract. This says Johnson, combined with some gentle exercises burns fat and tones muscles. Dr Robert Girandola, professor of Exercise Science at the University of Southern California is convinced that Oxycise can burn up calories. In a recent study, he found women burned 140 per cent more calories with Oxycise than riding an exercise bike. But many experts are sceptical of the evidence.

Whether Oxycise works or not deep breathing provides your body's cells with oxygen, which helps you absorb nutrients. It also stimulates your lymphatic system to get rid of toxins. If your breath is shallow, also known as chest breathing, your cells are receiving fewer nutrients and your lymph system may be more sluggish, both of which may lead to weight gain.

So get out into nature were the air is pure and fill your lungs with oxygen-rich air. It is the most natural thing you can do.

"When you arise in the morning, think of what a precious privilege it is to be alive - to breathe, to think, to enjoy, to love."
Marcus Aurelius

DAY 23 – GREEK YOGURT

"I go to great pains to find the best yogurt."
Ezra Koenig

Few foods pack as healthy a punch in such small serving sizes as Greek yogurt. It was a stable part of my weight loss program. Mixed with berries and covered with Linseed it made a delicious breakfast. But what is Greek yogurt? Greek yogurt is what you get when you take regular yogurt, place it in some fine mesh cloth, and allow some of the liquid in it—whey, to be more precise—to slowly drain out, resulting in a thicker yogurt with less moisture. The more concentrated the yogurt, the more concentrated the flavour. You need to be aware that there are no rules about what can and cannot be called 'Greek yogurt.' You need to read the ingredient label. The main ingredients should be milk and live active cultures with nothing added.

So how does 'Greek yogurt' help us in our quest to rapidly lose weight?

Greek yogurt contains almost twice the amount of protein found in standard yogurt, and significantly less sugar, which means that not only will you feel satisfied for a longer time (appetite suppression), but also protein possesses a higher thermic effect than any other macronutrient.

Greek yogurt helps prevent yeast infections, they also promote digestive health. Digestive bacteria are responsible for assisting with digestion and produce waste as a result. If these cultures are insufficient, digestive disturbances can occur. It is important to keep the cultures well stocked and in good shape, as these little bacteria do lots for your health.

Greek yogurt contains most of the essential bone-building nutrients, such as calcium, magnesium, phosphorus and Vitamin D. Cortisol is a hormone associated with stress, bringing about numerous ill effects ranging from high blood pressure to fat retention and more. Calcium can reduce the negative impact of too much cortisol, as it helps with blood vessel relaxation and also prevents excessive fat storage.

A little known fact is that Greek yogurt is rich in iodine, a trace mineral that most associate with seafood. If you dislike seafood, however, you're in luck, as Greek yogurt can be a suitable alternative. Iodine is necessary for supporting healthy metabolic function, helping you keep the weight off as well.

If I haven't sold you on 'Greek yogurt' yet consider this. Our gut has a nerve known as the Vagus, which tends to directly relay signals from the gut to the brain, and vice versa. This explains why anxiety can result in nervous stomach, but also how yoghurt can improve your wellbeing. By decreasing the incidence of you experiencing intestinal disorders, and even buffering the effect of cortisol, this nerve is able to transmit to the brain that calm has been achieved. In response, the brain produces more serotonin and calms itself. All from making your gut happy.

'Greek yogurt' can be consumed at any time during the day, even around the workout period, and before bed. Yogurt contains both whey and casein protein, supplying a mix of fast and slow digesting amino nutrition. So go get a quality 'Greek yogurt' and make sure you always have a supply in your refrigerator.

DAY 24 – AN APPLE A DAY

"An apple a day keeps the doctor away"
Old Celtic Proverb

As a boy at the bottom of the garden was the old orchard. The apple trees had long passed their days of fruitfulness. They were good for not much else than climbing and playing in and eventually, they became firewood. Many of the older farm and country houses had small orchards as apples played a vital role in the diet. They could be carefully stored in a cool attic after being picked and provided a source of fruit when nothing else would have been available.

Loaded with antioxidants, filling fibre and a host of vitamins and minerals, apples truly are a powerfully slimming superfood. Apples are naturally free of fat, cholesterol, and sodium and a low calorie, yet nutrient dense food. Apples are a great source of dietary fibre – with 5 grams in one medium-size fruit. The type of fibre found in apples is soluble fibre, which can help people feel fuller, longer. Several different variants of diets are based on eating an apple 15 – 30 minutes before you eat a meal. The evidence shows that this leads to fewer calories being consumed. As well as the obesity-fighting powers of apples a recent study from Washington State University researchers linked eating apples (and in particular, Granny Smith apples) to the prevention of disorders associated with obesity. The non-digestible compounds (fibre, polyphenols) and low carbohydrates in apples remain intact when they reach the colon, where they are fermented by bacteria, which then benefits the growth of good bacteria in the gut. Researchers believe the discovery could help prevent some obesity disorders, including low-grade, chronic inflammation that can lead to diabetes.

The Glycemic effect (GI level) assigns a value to carbohydrate-containing foods based on their effects on the blood glucose levels of human test subjects. Foods that rank high on a scale of one to 100 can raise blood sugar quickly and significantly. Foods that rank low on the scale have a slower, less marked effect on blood sugar. The GI values for the apples tested by the Glycemic Index Foundation range from 28 to 44. The type of apple, the ripeness of the fruit and other factors may affect its GI value, according to the American Diabetes Association. On average, this fruit falls into the lower end of the GI.

Not only is there only 47 calories in an average size apple but apples and many berries contain large amounts of pectin in their cell walls. Pectin encourages weight loss in that it helps to limit the amount of fat, cells can absorb. Pectin also has a water binding property that allows it to absorb watery substances and penetrate cells. These watery substances then bombard the cells and cause them to release fat deposits.

Crisp, juicy, full of sweet-sharp flavours and nutrition. Add to that the convenient portability and year-round availability, it's no wonder apples are enjoyed by many each and every day. Put all this together and it makes an apple the ideal snack to have at hand if no other healthy food can be found or as a planned snack in your daily eating plan.

DAY 25 – WEIGH YOURSELF

"I'm not there yet, but I'm closer than I was yesterday."
Anon

One of the key strengths of your weight loss goal is that it is easily measurable. Now like everything in life it can also be complicated but we are sticking to measuring a straightforward drop in your overall weight. A scale is a powerful tool. When you're losing weight, it's extremely satisfying to see those numbers go down. During my 40 days, I weighed myself at least once a day. You should pick a consistent time of day to weigh yourself as your weight fluctuates greatly throughout each and every day. I recommend that you step on the scales first thing in the morning and record your progress perhaps in an app as discussed earlier.

There are other interesting and motivational ways to track the progress of your weight loss journey. If like me you have piled on the pounds over the years with an ever-increasing waste line then you will also have made the sad journey to ever increasing clothes sizes. So select a pair of trousers or jeans that you have to make a little effort to get the zip up and buttons closed. Put them on and then leave a few days before you try again. It is a good, good feeling when you no longer have to struggle to get them on and then when they are actually becoming loose. Feeling more comfortable in your clothes or going down a size is even more important than the scale because they're more accurate signs of fat loss versus the fluid shifts you can see on the scale. Your body tells a story.

Once your old clothes get too loose and baggy let them go. Don't hold on to them 'just in case.' There is no going back, this is the new you. You got in shape because you wanted to feel and look different, so if you're favourite jeans or top simply doesn't fit anymore, see it as the positive it is. It's time for a new start, a new you, and yes, even some new clothes. Remember to donate your clothes to someone who can benefit from them.

Another way to track your weight loss is to take progress photos. The whole world is going selfie mad so we might as well join in. Take a photo of yourself — ideally wearing the same clothes, standing in the same position, and in the same place — once a week or every couple of weeks. This will help you see the changes you might not notice when you're looking at yourself every day.

Of course, the best way to find out that you are losing weight and the way that provides the greatest motivation to keep going is when people notice and remark on it. When you are greeted with a sincere 'hello you are looking well, have you lost weight?' brings great pleasure. This can't be bought or forced but is the reward of your perseverance and determination.

The common advice is not to weigh yourself every day but once a week or fortnight. The big problem with this is the temptation to cheat for a few days after your weigh-in and then panic in the day or two before your next weigh-in. Daily weighing keeps you focused during this intensive 40-day journey.

☐

DAY 26 – RISE AND SHINE

According to the rest of the world when we Irish meet each other in the morning we all say in our strong Irish brogues (accent) "top of the morning to you." In fact, I am not sure when last I heard someone use this expression. While this might be dated and stereotypical, it does contain a great truth. The expression is literally saying 'may the best of the morning be yours.' Morning in Ireland during the summer is certainly a wonderful time of the day, but not so great on a cold, dark winter's day. Getting up early in the morning helps you better deal with negativity and enhances your chances of success. According to Christopher Randler, a biology professor at the University of Education in Heidelberg, Germany, "When it comes to business success, morning people hold the important cards. My earlier research showed that they tend to get better grades in school, which get them into better colleges, which then lead to better job opportunities. Morning people also anticipate problems and try to minimize them. They're proactive. Many studies have linked this trait, proactivity, with better job performance, greater career success, and higher wages." It's not very surprising to know that some of the most successful people in the world are also early risers.

But how does it help you lose weight? Scientists have found that getting up early and enjoying the early morning light helps lower body fat because the 'blue light' of the morning kick-starts the body's metabolism. Even just 20-

30 minutes of morning sunlight is enough to keep off the pounds. It is thought that early morning light triggers certain genes which are linked to the internal body clock and kick-starts the metabolism. "Light is the most potent agent to synchronize your internal body clock that regulates circadian rhythms, which in turn also regulate energy balance," said study senior author Dr Phyllis Zee, Professor of Neurology at Northwestern University Feinberg School of Medicine.

The message is that you should get more bright light between 8 a.m. and mid-day. As part of a healthy lifestyle, we should be seeking to get more appropriate exposure to light. A study looked at 54 people of an average age of 30. They wore a wrist monitor that measured their light exposure and sleep parameters for seven days in normal-living conditions. Their caloric intake was determined from seven days of food logs. They found that those who were regularly exposed to more morning light had lower BMIs.

The morning is also a good time to prepare healthy meals for the day, rather than after work when your motivation levels are low and you are really tired. If you're not a morning person take baby steps. Start slowly by waking up earlier than you normally do, like 15 minutes for the first week, 20 minutes the following week, and so forth until you reach your goal time.

"As the olde englysshe prouerbe sayth in this wyse. Who soo woll ryse erly shall be holy helthy & zely."
The Book of St. Albans, printed in 1486:
Made popular by Benjamin Franklin as
"Early to bed and early to rise, makes a man healthy, wealthy and wise"

DAY 27 – LIFT SOMETHING HEAVY

Maybe it has dawned on you that we have got to day 27 and I haven't mentioned the gym (that is because I didn't go to the gym, maybe when I feel comfortable with my goal weight I might) or really any exercise (don't forget the walking, you've gotta move) but one thing will help you reach your goal. If you take a look inside a gym, you're likely to see people trying to lose weight and the "best" way they know how to accomplish this is by ramping up their time spent doing cardiovascular exercise. But, is this really the "best" way to lose weight? You could like me avoid the gym altogether and lift heavy things. Lifting weights give you an edge over belly fat, stress, heart disease, and cancer. Scientists found that being strong during middle age is associated with "exceptional survival," defined as living to the age of 85 without developing a major disease. Stronger people live longer, survive hardships better, and are able to enjoy life more fully than weaker people.

When Penn State researchers put dieters into three groups—no exercise, aerobic exercise only, or aerobic exercise and weight training—they all lost around 21 pounds, but the lifters shed six more pounds of fat than those who didn't pump iron. Why? The lifters' loss was almost pure fat; the others lost fat and muscle. Other research on dieters who don't lift shows that, on average, 75 percent of their weight loss is from fat, while 25 percent is from muscle. Muscle loss may drop your scale weight, but it doesn't improve your reflection in the mirror and it makes you more likely to gain back the flab you lost. However, if you weight train as you diet, you'll protect your hard-earned muscle and burn more fat. The more muscle you have the more energy the body requires even at rest.

Mark Sisson in the 'Primal Blueprint' recommends that you do "Two to three Lift Heavy Things workouts of 7-30 minutes each week." This is not hours pumping iron that we are talking about. Lifting heavy things makes bones strong. The bone acts (along with the muscle) as a lever during the lift, which places a lot of stress on the bone. To recover from the activity and be ready for the next time it has to fulfil lever duty, the bone remodels itself, gaining density and getting stronger and more durable. Movements that engage the whole body, like deadlifts and farmer carries, will be most effective and efficient. These exercises replicate real world movements. Pick up rocks, logs, concrete blocks, anything heavy ... then carry them to another place. Lift with your legs! Other workouts that I practised during my 40 days included Kettlebells, Burpees (check out YouTube if you're not sure how these work) and carrying a very fancy sandbag around.

Knowing you're strong, and feeling it too, feels amazing. And when you feel amazing, your outlook on life shifts, and you start to realise you can do amazing things.

"Go forth and lift heavy things..."
Mark Sisson

DAY 28 – WHAT COLOUR IS YOUR TEA?

Irish people are the second biggest tea drinkers in the world. Using data compiled by Euromonitor and the World Bank, Quartz calculates that we get through 4.8 lbs per head every year. That puts Ireland in second place globally, over half a pound ahead of the UK. Only Turkey get through more tea, with an astonishing seven pounds per head consumed there. Irish tea is far more than just a hot drink to go with your digestive biscuit, is an important Irish custom that serves as a symbol of hospitality, companionship, and friendship.

The Irish tea culture dates back to the 1800s when it was imported from English merchants. Irish tea was generally of cheaper quality so they added milk, sometimes as much as 1/3 of the cup, to cover up the taste. This meant that Irish tea had to be brewed stronger than its English counterpart and it still is to today. A proper cup of tea is brewed in a heated teapot until it is a dark colour, commonly known as a good strong cup of tea.

During my 40 day journey, I changed the colour of my tea to a more Irish green. Green tea has been gaining popularity in the West but for a long time, it has been used in traditional Chinese medicine to treat various conditions from headaches to healing wounds. Green tea has become a popular product associated with weight loss. It is claimed that green tea might help the body's metabolism be more efficient. Green tea contains caffeine and a type of flavonoid called catechin, which is an antioxidant. Research shows that both of these compounds can speed up metabolism. Catechin can also help to break down excess fat, while both catechin and caffeine can increase the amount of energy the body uses. A review published in 2010 stated that Catechins or an epigallocatechin gallate (EGCG)–caffeine mixture has a small positive effect on weight loss.

Catechin polyphenols in green tea also appear to stimulate the use of fatty acids by liver and muscle cells. This then reduces the rate that carbohydrates are used and allows for more endurance and longer exercise times. Green tea is also thought to lower Ghrelin levels. Ghrelin is often referred to as the 'hunger hormone'. If ghrelin is high, then you are hungrier. This might explain the claim that green tea reduces or suppresses hunger. Some people have claimed amazing results from drinking as much as twelve cups of green tea a day. It is important to note that any benefits of green tea for weight loss are likely to be very small.

Bottom line is this, tea, of whatever colour, is relaxing, pleasant to drink certainly unless you are consuming huge amounts of it will do you no harm and if it is coloured green it may just help you towards your weight loss goal.

"You can't get a cup of tea big enough or a book long enough to suit me."
C. S. Lewis

DAY 29 – THE HUNGER GAME

Salad might be "boring" when you're craving chocolate, but if you're truly hungry, it tastes amazing. Hunger is a powerful obstacle to weight loss because it is one of the most basic of human instincts. So many people find that hunger pangs becoming a stronger pull than their desire to lose weight. As they cut back on their food intake, their body starts calling out in hunger and they give in to that cry. The three most powerful human needs are Fluids, Feeding and Procreation. Hunger was and is an important survival mechanism for mankind. Controlling hunger is one of the keys to long-term weight loss. Most calorie restriction plans ignore this factor, pretending it is all about willpower. You can't 'decide' to be less hungry.

It is not wrong or bad to be hungry. Mild or moderate hunger is normal and is something that you should be experiencing three to four times a day. It is your bodies' way of saying that you have burned off the previous meal and it's time to fill up again for the hours ahead. If you are never really hungry it is a sure signal that you are eating too much and you are unlikely to lose weight. If you are carrying excess weight a little mild hunger will not hurt you. Better than that it might even make you feel invigorated and warrior-like. The key is not letting yourself get so hungry that it derails your weight loss strategy. You want to be able to be comfortable with hunger.

Try eating a smaller portion of a meal than you normally would and then don't snack between meals allowing yourself to get hungry. The advice to "eat when you're hungry; stop when you're full," is great wisdom, but it is meaningless if you don't know what hunger actually feels like. We put on weight by responding more to "brain hunger," cravings, emotions, boredom, social pressure etc. Particularly here in Ireland, meal times can be so set and established leading us to eat the food set in front of us whether we are hungry or not. When we learn if our body is truly hungry and then eat only enough nutritious food to satisfy that hunger we are well on our way to achieving weight loss.

When you feel hunger, don't eat immediately. Ponder the sensation and ask yourself the question is this really "body hunger" and not hunger that is coming from another source or stimulus, seeing or smelling something nice for instance. After a period of true hunger eat slowly and calmly the foods that you have chosen to eat. Remember to chew. Really enjoy the amazing taste and the sensation of satisfying your hunger. Mild hunger always makes your food that much better when it does come.

"Being hungry like a lion, enduring hunger for extended periods of time is not a bad thing. It is actually great for our health. It is also sometimes called – fasting. And including it to your healthy lifestyle will get you closer to becoming invincible."
Milan Stolicny

Please Note: If you're in recovery from an eating disorder, or if you have another medical problem that could make skipping meals dangerous, none of this applies to you.

DAY 30 – GO NUTS

A massive danger in your aim to lose weight rapidly over a relatively short period of time is that you give into the hunger cravings and go on a huge binge that leads to a downward spiral of overeating again. That is why it is important to have healthy snacks available that can curb your hunger pangs and stop you bingeing. Convenient, portable and that don't have to be eaten that day are important points to consider. That is why having an apple available is a good idea. Another food that falls into this category is nuts. Nuts are extremely healthy, as they're full of nutrients packed with protein, fibre, monounsaturated fats, vitamin E, folic acid, magnesium, copper, and antioxidants. They have been linked to a wide range of health benefits, including protection against heart disease and diabetes.

Although they are high in fat, it's unsaturated heart-healthy fats. The fact that they are high in calories and fat is the reason that many people avoid them, fearing that they are fattening but the scientific evidence does not back this up. Bad fats that pose health problems come primarily from saturated and trans fats, neither of which are found in most nuts. Instead, most nuts are loaded with good fats: -- monounsaturated and polyunsaturated fats. Some nuts, such as walnuts, boast a rich source of heart-healthy omega-3 fatty acids, similar to salmon.

A Purdue University study found that as counter-intuitive as it seems, the participants who ate 1.5 oz per day of lightly salted, dry roasted almonds (250 cal. worth) actually had less appetite throughout the day and didn't gain weight.

Not all nuts are created equal and some will help us on our weight loss journey more than others. Almonds contain good amounts of healthy fats that are useful for the body. They also contain a good amount of fibre that aids digestion of food and ensure a healthy bowel movement. Almonds have a high protein which can help develop a lean muscle mass. The mono-unsaturated fats maintain and reduce our body mass index.

Walnuts are nutrient dense foods, power-packed with minerals like manganese and copper. It also contains an antioxidant compound known as ellagic acid that helps to block metabolic processes like inflammation that may lead to insulin resistance and diabetes. Walnuts help lose weight; thanks to the presence of omega-3 fatty acids, protein and fibre that make you feel satiated, hence leaving you not craving for lesser foods.

Pistachios or pistas are high in fibre content, which keeps you fuller for longer, thus preventing over-eating. The fibre present in this nut also helps in boosting metabolism. Moreover, the soluble mono-unsaturated fats in pista may help prevent weight gain.

Warning: Don't go too nuts. The key is portion control. Nuts, in general, are calorie dense—160-200 calories per ounce—enjoy in moderation. Pre-portion nuts in small bags. They are a great snack to take on the go or to the office. Choose nuts in the shell; you will probably eat fewer since it takes time to crack them.

> *"The combined results of four huge studies, including more than 170,000 men and women, show that munching on nuts on all or most days of the week cuts the risk of heart attack by an incredible 35 percent."*
> The Healthy Heart Miracle Diet

Make sure you are not allergic to nuts as it may trigger serious health problems.

DAY 31 - MOTIVATE YOURSELF

"You wouldn't worry so much about what others think of you if you realized how seldom they do."
Eleanor Roosevelt

A sad reality is that we live in a world that tends towards the negative rather than the positive. If this is not your experience great, but for many unfortunately it will be. This simply means that you need to motivate and encourage yourself. We don't want to dwell on the negativity that may come your way from what my son calls 'the haters,' but to power on in positivity towards the weight that you have visualised at your goal end.

Being motivated to lose weight is important for long-term weight loss success. If you have no one cheering you on then you must practice personal tough love. Keep reading and writing out your goals, keep picturing that end result, keep pressing towards the finish line. Keep reading through this book putting into practice the hints along the way.

Ideally, it is great if you have someone to walk this journey with you, holding each other accountable and encouraging each other throughout the process. If you have no immediate support group like a weight loss buddy or a support group that you can attend then think about finding an online support system. There are various online support groups that you can join on social media that you might find helpful. Having strong social support will help hold you accountable and keep you motivated to lose weight.

Motivate yourself by establishing a reward system. We are hardwired for positive reinforcement, so giving yourself healthy rewards along the way can be really good for your weight loss motivation. (As long as you're not rewarding yourself with a binge day of chocolate, junk food and ice-cream after a week of healthy eating.) Break your big goal into weekly goals and each time you reach one of these steps on the ladder give yourself a reward. You don't have to spend a lot of money, just put some little rewards in place to motivate you along the way. Some of my rewards were simply being able to wear comfortably clothes that I hadn't been able to put on for years. Try to make your reward an activity or experience rather than food or drink.

My biggest motivation during my 40 days was seeing the scales tick downwards day after day. I knew that if I had been disciplined in my diet and faithful in my walking exercise program following the helps that I am writing about that when I went on the scales in the morning that I would be delighted with the result. It was brilliant to face the scales with excitement rather than dread. I hope that this is your experience too. Remember that even if you haven't been a perfect dieter you are still making progress towards your end goal.

"Don't wait until everything is just right. It will never be perfect. There will always be challenges, obstacles, and less than perfect conditions. So what? Get started now. With each step you take, you will grow stronger and stronger, more and more skilled, more and more self-confident, and more and more successful."
Mark Victor Hansen

DAY 32 – DIET DRINKS

Despite claims that the consumption of sugary drinks may lead to an estimated 184,000 adult deaths each year worldwide, the soda industry is still a $75-billion market. So many diets that I have read, have an easy answer to this problem, diet drinks that use artificial sweeteners like aspartame. I'm talking about Diet Coke, (other brands are available) sugar-free sweets and mints, and even desserts. Aspartame tastes pretty decent. It's sweet, and it really does have zero calories. But at what cost?

Instead of sugar, manufacturers load up diet drinks with aspartame and other artificial sweeteners to give that sugary taste without the calories. The problem is that these sweeteners can be more deadly than actual sugar. Diet sodas have actually been shown to lead to weight gain. A study, listed by the American Diabetes Association, has shown a link between consuming diet sodas and having an increased waist size. In fact, those who drank diet sodas actually had a waist size of up to 70% greater than non-drinkers.

There are over 92 documented side effects of artificial sweeteners. Here are 12 of the more common effects: *impaired vision *tinnitus (ringing or buzzing in ears) *noise intolerance *epileptic seizures *migraines *memory loss *fatigue *depression *anxiety *insomnia *phobias *weight gain

In case you missed it, read that last one again: weight gain. Let me try and explain why this happens. It is due to what is called the cephalic phase response of the brain. This causes a conditioned reflex that is well established as a result of a lifelong experience with a sweet taste that is associated with the introduction of new energy into the body. When sweet taste stimulates the tongue, the brain programs the liver to prepare for the arrival of new energy, sugar, from outside. The liver, in turn, stops the manufacture of sugar from the protein and starch reserves of the body and instead begins to store the metabolic fuels that are circulating in the blood. If it is sugar entering the body then the liver is doing its proper job of regulation. But if the sweet taste is not followed by sugar nutrient availability, then the body will have an urge to eat. The more sweet taste that runs over our tongue without the actual accompanying calories the more urge there is to eat and overeat. This urge to eat can last up to 90 minutes after you consume the diet drink.

Can I make this as simple as I can as I know and see so many thinking that by taking sugar substitutes that it helps them lose weight? You drink your artificially sweetened drink. Your tongue responds to the sweet taste, telling the brain, sugar is coming. Your brain tells your liver and your body prepares for the sugar then no sugar comes. This leads your body to start crying out sugar, give me sugar. This leads to the urge to eat in order that the body can get the sugar that it thought was coming. And the food your body will be craving is the most sugar-laden that it can imagine.

Our whole aim is to get our mind and body working for us in weight loss not against us, so please, no artificial sweeteners in drinks or anything else we consume.

> *"The fact that sweeteners fatten people is generally well known.... sweeteners also poison your metabolism so you cannot burn calories."*
> Jane Bowen, M.D.

DAY 33 – SPRINT

"I just give everything I've got irrespective of what the circumstances may be."
Elon Musk

If you are following my advice you are everyday walking, walking and walking a little bit more. Now we are going to ramp it up slightly and add in a little sprinting. Exercise physiologist Martin Gibala from McMaster University has found that 1 minute of intense exercise is all you need to get the same benefits of a more moderate 45-minute session. "Brief bursts of intense exercise are remarkably effective" she found. If you want to boost health and fitness and you don't have 45 minutes or an hour to work out, our data show that you can get big benefits from even a single minute of intense exercise.

Studies have shown that while regular exercise can add six years to your life. That benefit can disappear once you're clearing more than 48 km (30 miles) per week. Instead of running long endurance distances keep walking and add in some sprints. Try wind sprints - If you live near a hill (it doesn't have to be terribly steep; any incline works), walk or jog to it to warm up. Sprint up it for 20 seconds. Rest while you walk back down. Repeat at least three times (for a challenge, work up to six-plus sprints). At three sets, this will take you a total of only five to seven minutes. Try this two or three times a week and you will get results.

Sprint intervals improve insulin sensitivity. Sprinting increases the oxidative (fat burning) potential of muscle and improves endurance capacity. It also improves the efficiency of muscle during exercise, so you can conserve more glycogen and rely on more fat. It's even an effective way to improve agility and speed.

There just might also be some psychology behind this. Jon Gabriel of 'The Gabriel Method' says, "There's a reason for this, and it's something I've been talking about for years. I call it the 'get thin or get eaten' body adaptation." Imagine in the environment where you live there are predators that are capable of eating you, and every once in a while one of them came out and chased you. If you weren't lightning fast for 10, 20, 30 seconds, and outran everybody else, you were dead. And if you are faster than everybody else in a 10-second sprint or a 20-second sprint, you will survive. That is called short-term acute stress. Short-term acute stresses have differing effects on the body than long-term, chronic, low-grade stresses. It reverses hormonal problems like leptin and insulin resistance. They make your body more sensitive to these very important fat-regulating hormones, and it makes it much easier to lose weight.

If you had to run away from a predator that was intent on eating you, your body would get the message very quickly that if you weren't fast you were dead, and you activate what Jon Gabriel calls 'the get thin or get eaten adaptation.'

So go on, Sprint flat out for all your worth and as you are doing it try to vividly imagine a wild wolf, bear or whatever your nearest predator might be trying to catch you for its dinner. See if your body gets the message.

"Run, Forrest, run!"
Jenny Curran

DAY 34 – PREPARE YOUR OWN FOOD

"If you want to prioritize health, you're going to have to prioritize cooking and develop a relationship with your kitchen. Boxes won't provide you with what you need."
Dr. Yoni Freedhoff, author of The Diet Fix.

If you were alive then, think back to what life was like in the 1970s. Obesity, unlike today, was scarce: In a classroom full of 30 children, it was statistically likely that only one would be obese. People weren't obsessed with working out and the latest diet book. The reason why everyone was so slim didn't have anything to do with exercise machines or diet supplements they just ate a lot of home cooking free from added sugars, salt and saturated fat.

Preparing food from scratch makes us healthier however it's easier than ever not to cook at home. Press a few buttons on your app or make a phone call and food arrives at your door. But that convenience can come at a high-calorie cost. One simple, and usually less expensive, way to stop those extra calories from heading for your waistline? Cook at home.

In a recent study of more than 18,000 people, University of Illinois researchers reported that when dining out, people ate 190 more calories per meal than they did at home. That amounts to over 50,000 calories in a year - the equivalent of 14 lbs of fat. They also took in more saturated fat and sodium—both shown in other studies to wreck your metabolism and encourage weight gain. The shocking result is that restaurant meals had almost as much fat and even more sodium than fast-food meals.

Jean-Michel Cohen believes he has the cure for obesity. If we want to lose weight, Cohen says, we should cook more meals. Cohen, whose book, The Parisian Diet, has sold more than two million copies states that societies that cook more meals are slimmer and healthier. Like the French, for instance. Only 16.9 per cent of the French population are obese, compared to 22.7 per cent of people in the UK, who cook far less than the French, and 33.9 per cent of Americans, who cook even less.

One of the biggest problems is the lack of time. Starting to cook a meal from scratch takes considerable more time than convenience food. The key to cooking at home is knowing what you are going to cook. Plan the menu for a week, shop once and prepare some foods ahead of time. Clean and chop fresh vegetables so they're ready for meals and snacks.

It is also important to cook food in a healthy oil as oil plays an important role in your health and wellness. Coconut oil is one of the healthiest cooking oils which help you lose weight and burn belly fat. Coconut oil does not contain sodium, cholesterol or carbohydrates. By adding coconut oil to your diet, you will increase the amount of healthy fats that you are giving your body. Coconut oil also helps your body absorb fat-soluble vitamins.

Leave the packaged or bought meals to one side. Plan a healthy meal, buy some fresh ingredients, cook and enjoy.

DAY 35 – EAT FAT TO LOSE FAT

Eating fat does not make you fat, argues a new report by the National Obesity Forum (NOF) and the Public Health Collaboration, as they demanded a major overhaul of official dietary guidelines. The report says the low-fat and low-cholesterol message, which has been official policy in the UK since 1983, was based on "flawed science" and had resulted in an increased consumption of junk food and carbohydrates.

For years Dr Mark Hyman was a vegetarian who kept his intake of dietary fat to a minimum. Whole-wheat bread, grains, beans, pasta and fruits and vegetables made up the bulk of his diet, just as the government's dietary guidelines had long recommended. But as he got older, Dr Hyman noticed something that bothered him: Despite plenty of exercise and a seemingly healthy diet, he was gaining weight and getting flabby. At first, he wrote it off as a normal part of ageing. But then he made a shift in his diet, deciding to eat more fat, not less – and the changes he saw surprised him. He lost weight, his love handles disappeared, and he had more energy. He encouraged his patients to consume more fat as well, and many of them lost weight and improved their cholesterol. Some even reversed their Type 2 diabetes.

This runs contrary to popular diet wisdom that preaches fat makes us fat. Research shows that actually, the right fats can help you become fit and healthy. Always remember that it is sugar, not fat that is the real thief stealing our health and affecting our waistlines. Fat is complex. We have saturated, monounsaturated, polyunsaturated and even Trans fats. Some fats are good; others neutral; and yes, some are bad.

A review of all the research on saturated fat published in the American Journal of Clinical Nutrition found no correlation between saturated fat and heart disease. Trans fat and inflammatory vegetable oils are unhealthy and play a role in chronic disease. However, consuming omega 3s are good for us. Healthy cell walls made from high-quality fats are better able to metabolize insulin, which keeps blood sugar better regulated. Fat also helps with stress management, cognition, mood, sleep, energy, weight management, healthy tissues, skin and hair – even digestion and nutrient absorption.

Your brain is about 60 percent fat. Of that percentage, the biggest portion comes from the omega-3 fat called docosahexaenoic acid (DHA). Your brain needs DHA to spark communication between cells. Easy access to high-quality fat boosts cognition, happiness, learning and memory. In contrast, studies link a deficiency of omega-3 fatty acids to depression, anxiety, bipolar disorder and schizophrenia.

The higher-quality the fat, the better your body will function. That's because the body uses the fat you eat to build cell walls. You have more than 10 trillion cells in your body and every single one of them needs high-quality fat. Just like your body needs nutrients from carbohydrates your body also requires fat in order to function properly. Eating fat is part of a balanced diet giving you the nutrients your body needs to function properly.

"Eat fat to get slim. Don't fear fat; fat is your friend."
Dr Malhotra

DAY 36 – FOCUS ON BEING HEALTHY RATHER THAN THIN

"Good health and good sense are two of life's greatest blessings."
Publilius Syrus

If you are overweight you are probably unhealthy. Studies show that when someone is categorized as obese, the likelihood of them being fit is very low. Being obese generally means lower fitness. But the reality is that you can be thinner and also unhealthy. That is why we have sought to place a strong emphasis on eating healthy nutritious foods throughout this book. We want to feed our body the right stuff so that it doesn't crave the wrong stuff (sugar and processed food). Processed foods usually have all the fibre stripped out and sugar and salt are added. Our bodies operate the best when we eat whole foods. Whole foods are foods found in their most natural state. Being healthy is all about eating natural food from the farm instead of the factory. The next time you are faced with a food choice ask yourself "Which choice is more about being healthy?"

Being fit and healthy is more than what you look like on the outside, we have to take care of our overall well-being too. It's important to remember that how you look in the mirror or the number on the scale shouldn't be your only incentive. A desire to lose weight should be first and foremost motivated by the need to be healthy. During my weight loss journey, there were different times that I began to notice changes that weren't reflected by the scales. In the morning I never had what I called 'rumbly guts,' from eating too much of the wrong kind of food the night before. I began to feel stronger and have more energy. I was able to walk further and faster than I could before. I knew that my body was changing for the better and that encouraged me to keep on going.

Siri Steinmo, a health psychology practitioner and personal trainer who designs 'antidiet' weight management courses, says our obsessive focus on being thin has displaced any focus on health. Living healthy is about more than shedding pounds; it's about treating your body right, strengthening muscles and feeding it the nutrients it needs for optimal function. Your mental and emotional health is also of vital importance. If thinness is your life's goal, you're going to end up pretty one-dimensional. It's good to try to be slim but not at the expense of everything else in your life. It's not about what you look like but what you can do with your body and mind that matters!

Ultimately, you really are what you eat, and having a bad diet is not good for you. It can lead to decreased strength, performance, reduced immunities and accelerated ageing. A key is to concentrate on what we are doing to take care of our inside more than what we look like on the outside. Focus on living a healthier, more active lifestyle and measuring your success not only by what you see on the scale but also with how energized and comfortable you feel within your own body.

"It's to change both how I look and how I feel that has motivated me to change what I eat."
- Chris Froome

DAY 37 – YOU CAN DO IT! LEARNED HELPLESSNESS

"Learned helplessness is the giving-up reaction, the quitting response that follows from the belief that whatever you do doesn't matter."
Arnold Schwarzenegger

Wow, you are nearly at the end of this book. If you have read right through to here, thank you. It means so much to me that the helps, hints and hacks that transformed my body and life have the ability to make such a difference to you also.

As I went through this process I was struck with a fear. What if someone reads the book, thinks about the content, has a need and desire to lose weight, and then goes, "I don't think that I can." Perhaps this comes from past failures and leaves you thinking, "I can't change, it is a waste of time trying, I just have to accept the way that I am." This is what psychologists call 'Learned Helplessness.'

In 1965 a man by the name of Martin Seligman did an unethical experiment to try and reverse what Pavlov had done with his dogs. He would ring a bell and then instead of giving the dog a treat, he would give it a light electric shock. After a number of times, the dog reacted to the shock even before it happened. As soon as the dog heard the bell, it reacted as though it already had been shocked.

But, then something unexpected happened. Seligman put

Thinking About Losing Weight

each dog into a large crate that was divided down the middle with a low fence. The dog could see and jump over the fence if necessary. The floor on one side of the fence was electrified, but not on the other side of the fence. Seligman put the dog on the electrified side and administered a light shock. He expected the dog to jump to the non-shocking side of the fence. Instead, the dogs lay down. It was as though they'd learned from the first part of the experiment that there was nothing they could do to avoid the shocks, so they gave up in the second part of the experiment.

Seligman described their condition as learned helplessness, or not trying to get out of a negative situation because the past has taught you that you are helpless. The problem is people can be just like these dogs. If over the course of your life, you have experienced crushing defeat or pounding abuse or loss of control, you learn over time to helplessly accept your situation. Learned helplessness is a natural response. "I have tried and failed so I am just not going to try again." By giving up we are saving ourselves from the pain of potential future failure. The more times we have given up the less likely we are to try again.

If that is the way you feel I want you to think about this. Your helplessness has been learned, therefore it can be unlearned. You are not destined to be overweight and suffer from all the associated health problems that go with it. You can learn to change. Please read to the end of the book. Then if you didn't do it go back to the start and do the Why and SMART goal exercises, follow the advice and begin to walk towards a new healthier, fitter you. You can overcome this way of experiencing life; the past does not have to dictate your present or future. Please keep reading.

DAY 38 – YOU CAN DO IT! SELF-EFFICACY

At its most basic, learned helplessness is believing you can't, self-efficacy is believing you can. To give a more expansive definition, self-efficacy is the belief in one's capabilities to organize and execute the courses of action required to manage prospective situations. It is your belief in your own ability to get it done. It is the difference between taking a passive position of defeat and the active position of facing a challenge. Whatever you learn can be unlearned. You can override your thoughts, limits and perceptions.

So how do we develop self-efficacy? The first way is through positive experiences. The more you experience success in reaching your goals the greater your sense that you can keep on doing it. In many ways, if you are very overweight this makes it easy as the first few excess pounds can be amongst the easiest to lose. Then when you see them dropping off it gives you the self-believe that you can keep on going towards your goal.

Another way is by seeing others succeed. Seeing people similar to yourself succeed by sustained effort raises your belief that you can do it too. For years a relative of mine struggled with being overweight. She blamed it on a medical condition. But when she made the decision to stop making excuses and start making changes she rapidly lost a considerable amount of weight. I am now at a weight that I haven't been for over 15 years. For the last 12 or so of those years, I have been trying and thinking about losing weight. Through what I have shared with you I have

Thinking About Losing Weight

stopped trying and started doing and yes with effort but with little pain have achieved my weight loss goal and you can too.

When you focus on things you have no control over, it can lead you to feel hopeless to change your situation. So, instead of doing that – focus on the things you can control. If you feel your situation is totally hopeless, begin with small changes. Cut out the sugary drinks and the crisps, sweets and chocolates. Take a small step and seek to maintain that first. That alone could make a big difference in your weight. You have the ability to make the right choices. Also, try to look at your situation in the most positive way you can. Count your blessings, all the good things you have going for you and believe that things will get better. Tell yourself, "I can do something about this." Then begin to make changes in your diet and lifestyle.

Remember people experience setbacks and failures every day and yet they pick themselves back up and keep trying. No matter how bad the past has been I believe you can be one of those people. Even the smallest positive change that you make is better than sitting in helplessness. The difference between being a victim and being a battling underdog is all about mind-set. Don't lie-down waiting for the shock but jump the fence to a new, confident, thinner and healthier you.

"People who have a sense of self-efficacy bounce back from failure; they approach things in terms of how to handle them rather than worrying about what can go wrong."
Albert Bandura

DAY 39 – YOU ARE AMAZING

"The human body and mind are tremendous forces that are continually amazing scientists and society. Therefore, we have no choice but to keep an open mind as to what the human being can achieve."
Evelyn Glennie

You are a walking, living breathing miracle. Don't allow yourself to be ground down by the cruel circumstances of life. Lift up your head and push through whatever obstacles there might be in your way. Don't let anything stop you from becoming the best possible you. Have you ever stopped to ponder how awesome your body is? In AsapSCIENCE's latest video, "Why Your Body Is AMAZING!" hosts Mitchell Moffit and Gregory Brown explain the human body consists of seven octillion atoms, making up the 37 trillion cells in our body, which can regenerate themselves over time.

The cells that line the stomach, regenerate every five days, which makes sense since stomach acid can dissolve metal. Meanwhile, the skin's outer layer, known as the epidermis, sheds every two to four weeks (roughly 1.5 pounds per year) of dead skin. On the other hand, some cells have been with us our entire lives, specifically those of the inner lens of the eyes, the muscle cells of the heart, and the neurons of the cerebral cortex in the brain (responsible for our memory).

When it comes to our sight, although we spend 10 percent of the day blinking, our eyes can actually distinguish between 2.3 to 7.5 million colours. In fact, studies have shown that after viewing 2,500 images for only three seconds, participants could recall if they had seen one of the images with 92 percent accuracy. This is contrary to the belief that long-term memory is not capable of storing images with detail.

Our touch and grasp, along with our sight, help us pinch and grab objects with our thumb, using the index and middle finger. However, it is the ring and pinky that gives us the ultimate hand power. When we put our hands together, we capture roughly the size of our heart as it beats 100,000 times a day, pumping 5.5 litres with each pulse, which is close to 3 million litres of blood every year. If a person were to live to 75, it would fill 90 Olympic size swimming pools.

Your DNA which is unique to you is supercoiled. If you stretched the DNA in one cell all the way out, it would be about 2m long and all the DNA in all your cells put together would be about twice the diameter of the Solar System. I could keep going describing how awesome you are.

When you consider what an amazing individual you are, surely you have an obligation to yourself, your family and the world at large to feed it the best nutrition you can, to give it the exercise it needs and to achieve your optimal weight. Chase your dreams, and live a life that's filled with passion and purpose.

"You made all the delicate, inner parts of my body and knit me together in my mother's womb. Thank you for making me so wonderfully complex! Your workmanship is marvellous—how well I know it."
The Psalmist, King David

DAY 40 – THE LAST LAUGH

"Laughter is important, not only because it makes us happy, it also has actual health benefits. And that's because laughter completely engages the body and releases the mind. It connects us to others, and that in itself has a healing effect."
Marlo Thomas

A 2006 study in the International Journal of Obesity found that laughing for 15 minutes each day can help you burn 10 to 40 calories, depending on your body size and the intensity of your laughter. This adds up to about one to four pounds of fat lost per year. That may not sound like much, but there's also been plenty of research linking happy people to all-around healthier lifestyles. In my weight loss experience, I have found that it has brought me moments of great pleasure along the way.

Forget the thought of daily battling cravings living a miserable life missing the sugar-filled things that used to bring you such pleasure. Focus on the new, the things that the thinner, healthier, fitter you can do that the old you could not accomplish. In the last week of my 40 days, I climbed a steep mountain with my teenage son. Now I did have to tell him to slow down a few times but for the most of the walk, I was able to keep up with him. We created some wonderful memories as we conquered that mountain together.

Hopefully, you read day 27 on lifting heavy things. I had two main weights, a 10 Kg Kettlebell and a 10 Kg sandbag. Three-quarters of the way through my journey I was doing some calculations on how much weight I had lost. You will have noticed that here in Ireland we still work in Stones and pounds when it comes to body weight. As I was converting my weight loss into Kgs this simple but profound reality struck me hard. I had lost more body weight than the 10 Kg Kettlebell that I had been using. In fact, when I reached my 40 lb goal I had nearly lost two of them. The day I reached my goal I took a photo of the equivalent of my weight loss – My 10 Kg Kettlebell, a 5 Kg Dumbbell and a 3 Kg Dumbbell. 18 Kgs in total. You can see that picture on my author page on Amazon.

If I had one message that I could impress on every overweight person this is it. Work out how much extra weight you are carrying then convert that into the equivalent of 10 Kg weights. Take one or two of those weights and go for a walk. Think of the fact that this is what you are dragging around with you every day all day. Walk with those weights until you can walk no further, set them down and then walk a little more without them. Feel the liberation and freedom and ease that it is now to walk without carrying the extra weight. That my friend is the greatest pleasure that my weight loss has brought me. More than the clothes I can now wear, more than the attention and admiration that my weight loss has brought, more than the renewed confidence that I now daily feel.

Expressed negatively it helped me realize the danger and damage of that extra weight. The strain that it must put on my heart and joints. Just the sheer fact of having to carry it all the time. Positively, now it is gone. Is it any wonder I have a skip in my step and a smile on my face. If you have read this far and are still 'Thinking about losing weight' still wondering if it is worth the effort, try it. Get a weight or something equivalent and carry it around. Think of that extra body weight and what effect it is having on you every day. Picture what life would be like with it gone and then resolve to go for it. Go back to the start of the book and develop your Why and your SMART goal and then stop thinking and start doing.

If you have begun to walk this weight loss journey or perhaps even this is you at the end of 40 days of putting these hints, helps and hacks into practice can I say a big **CONGRATULATIONS**. Every pound of weight gone is one pound that you don't have to carry around all day. Every step towards your goal is a success. There is no failure for today is a new day, just keep going. 40 days, 80 days, 160 days it does not matter, if you persevere you will accomplish your goal and reap the benefits and freedom that comes with it.

I used the information in this book to achieve my 40 lbs in 40 days of weight loss. Over 15 years of obesity, many failed attempts and then SUCCESS. I know that if I can do it so can you. Your weight loss doesn't have to be as rapid or dramatic as mine. Remember all weight loss if you are overweight is good, healthy and beneficial. If by reading this book I have helped you in some way to becoming healthier and happier then I have accomplished my goal.

I want to leave you with an ancient Irish Blessing entitled – "May the Road rise up to meet you." By way of explanation, it is about God's blessing for your journey. In Irish, the first line "Go n-éirí an bóthar leat" is more literally translated as "May you succeed on the road" the French equivalent of which is "bon voyage." May the road rise up to meet you means may your walk be an easy one - with no huge mountains to climb or obstacles to overcome. It alludes to three images from nature - the wind, sun and rain - as pictures of God's care and provision. For something written so long ago, the ancient Irish's deep connection to nature and Ireland's ever-changing elements shine through. The "wind" can be likened to the Spirit of God, who came as a "mighty wind" at Pentecost. The suns warmth in the prayer reminds us of the tender mercies of God, "by which the rising sun will come to us from heaven" (Gospel of Luke 1:78), whilst the soft falling rain speaks of God's provision and sustenance. Finally, we are reminded that we are held safe in God's loving hands as we travel on our journey through life when we trust Him with every situation.

May the road rise up to meet you.
May the wind be always at your back.
May the sun shine warm upon your face;
the rains fall soft upon your fields
and until we meet again,
may God hold you in the palm of His hand.

(Traditional Irish blessing)

ABOUT THE AUTHOR

James A. Love, also known as the Irish Guru, was born and has lived most of his life on the beautiful green island of Ireland. A practising life coach he has a passion to help as many people as he can, not just in his native land but right across the world, reach their potential in becoming the person that they were designed to be.

Check him out at:

www.irishguru.com

Printed in Great Britain
by Amazon